D1478447

SYPHILIS, PURITANISM AND WITCH HUNTS

Syphilis, Puritanism and Witch Hunts

Historical Explanations in the Light of Medicine and Psychoanalysis with a Forecast about Aids

Stanislav Andreski
Professor of Comparative Sociology
Polish University in London

St. Martin's Press   New York

306.461
A56a

© Stanislav Andreski 1989

First published in the United States of America in 1989

Printed in Hong Kong

ISBN 0–312–02702–8

KP

Library of Congress Cataloging-in-Publication Data
Andreski, Stanislav.
   Syphilis, Puritanism, and witch hunts : historical explanations in
the light of medicine and psychoanalysis with a forecast about AIDS /
Stanislav Andreski.
      p.   cm.
   Includes index.
   ISBN 0–312–02702–8 : $39.95
   1. Syphilis—Social aspects—History—16th century.
   2. Witchcraft—History—16th century.   I. Title.
   RA644.V4A65   1989
   306.4'61—dc20   89–31763
                                                              CIP

Contents

List of Illustrations

'Off to the Sabbat' by Queverdo
'The Four Witches' by Albert Durer

Foreword

The explanatory thesis presented here was published in a briefer form as articles in *Encounter*. I thank its editor for agreeing in advance to their re-publication in a book. These articles have been revised and expanded. The bulkiest addition, however, consists of the extracts from treatises on demonology which furnish additional support for my arguments.

The appendices have not been published before. They do not affect the explanatory thesis but deal with questions which arise from it. The first appendix has a direct bearing on the present situation as it contains a forecast of the social impact of Aids in the light of the history of older diseases. The second deals with more abstract problems and may be skipped by a reader uninterested in philosophy and comparative sociology.

It is a piece of good luck that the extracts from the sources are not only instructive but also amusing.

Part One
The Thesis

1

Syphilis, Puritanism and Capitalism

Emile Durkheim's methodological rule that social phenomena must be explained in terms of other social phenomena was a useful corrective to the abuse of biological analogies in the sociology of his time. But as a rigidly applied limitation it is just as obscurantist as the superstition about 'the mode of production' as the final and irreducible cause of everything else. In the light of knowledge available today we might find the views of Montesquieu and Adam Ferguson on the influence of climate too simplistic; but it would be absurd to deny that climate affects the culture. Recently the ecological movement has drawn our attention to the various ways in which pollution might put an end to progress. A well-supported thesis (by Derek Bryce-Smith, Professor of Chemistry at Reading University) has been put forward that lead poisoning is an important factor in the causation of juvenile delinquency. Here, accepting Weber's thesis that the puritanical ingredients of Protestantism constituted an essential factor in the development of capitalism, I shall try to trace the causation further back and inquire into the effects of another factor which might have constituted an equally crucial link, and which is neither religious nor economic but medical.

In his recent pioneering masterpiece, *Plagues and People*,[1] the Chicago historian William McNeill has been able to explain a number of turning points of history which hitherto appeared as inexplicable. The Spaniards' extraordinary success in conquering central and southern America – and, even more, the unparalleled rapidity of the conversion of the Indians – lose their miraculous character in the light of what McNeill tells us about the impact of the diseases (above all, smallpox and measles) brought from Europe. It seems justifiable to surmise that, seeing how they were succumbing to the disease which spared the Spaniards or at least afflicted them much less, the Indians would feel that their gods had either abandoned them or been overpowered by the mightier

3

god of the Spaniards. I want to put forward the view that the importation of syphilis into Europe had equally profound effects on European civilisation: affecting most directly religion and sexual morality, and indirectly economic development.

In one of his essays D. H. Lawrence attributes the rise of puritanism to the arrival of syphilis in Europe. As might be expected from a novelist, he confines himself to a brief affirmation without backing it with more systematic arguments. I believe that Lawrence is right and that his contention can be supported on three grounds: chronological congruence; psychological plausibility; and the complete inadequacy of alternative explanations.

I must stress the limits of my thesis: I do not attribute the Reformation as a whole to the impact of syphilis. Throughout the Middle Ages there have been heresies and outbursts of opposition to the Church and especially the Papacy. The consolidation of the royal power, the emergence of educated lay officials and lawyers, the growth of the cities and the proliferation of wealthy merchants, all created stronger counterweights to the power of the Church, weakened by disorder and corruption at the centre and the licentiousness and greed of the clergy. The increasing burden of ecclesiastical exactions evoked hostility and resistance among the peasants and townsmen, while the nobility coveted the constantly growing wealth of the Church. The spread of literacy and the invention of printing undermined the priests' monopoly of access to the Holy Writ. The Nordic nations' resentment at being exploited by the Italians and the Spaniards, who controlled the Church, also played a part in the complex causation sketched above.

If a medical factor was involved, it was probably the plague which preceded the Reformation, and which might have undermined the people's trust in the power of the priests to protect them. It is difficult, however, to imagine a mental process which would link the abhorrence of pleasure with the plague which, true enough, was commonly regarded as God's punishment for sins in general, but was not believed to be caused by enjoyment of carnal pleasures, as was the case with syphilis.

My thesis purports to explain not *all* the aspects of Protestantism or even Puritanism in the more general sense, but only the injection into them of puritanism in the sense of abhorrence of pleasures of the flesh – which includes comfort and repose, as well as the gratifications of bed and table. It is true, of course, that the ideals of asceticism drew a large number of practitioners throughout the

Christian past, but these were hermits, monks, nuns and to a lesser extent priests. During the sixteenth and seventeenth centuries, however, a milder but more effective form of renunciation began to affect a much larger part of the Christian populations. This process cannot be explained by the fortuitous emergence of prophets of genius – although we must not disregard *a priori* the importance of accidental causes – because preachers of asceticism have always abounded. What demands explanation is why more people became inclined to follow such teachings.

All forms of Protestantism had a much stronger puritanical streak than can be found in Catholicism with the exception of the monastic orders. In the latter denomination, asceticism was mainly for the monks, while for the laity faith was regarded as more important than behaviour. The institution of confession permitted ever renewed reconciliation of recidivist sinning with staunch faith. At the price of diminishing people's ability to enjoy life, the Protestant churches succeeded in imposing more effectively on the majority of their faithful, as well as on the entirety of their clergy (naturally with a few exceptions), a stricter code of behaviour in financial dealings and attitudes to work, and above all in all matters relating to sex. We must remember, however, that the Counter-Reformation also included a trend towards puritanism in the sense of the more rigorous enforcement of sexual morality inside the Catholic Church. Never afterwards can we find brazenly licentious Popes (like the Borgias) or monasteries where open fornication was the rule.

It seems exceedingly likely that the spread of puritanism was mainly due to the arrival of syphilis in Europe. Causation of great historical processes is always bafflingly complex, and clearly many other factors were involved. But this seems to me less uncertain than any other explanation: puritanism would not have had the appeal which helped it to find adherents so quickly and widely without the spread of syphilis.

This thesis fits the chronology: syphilis appeared shortly after the discovery of America, presumably brought to Europe by the sailors of Columbus' *Santa Maria*, in 1492, *i.e.* seventeen years before the birth of Calvin. According to Howard W. Haggard, Dr Roderic Diaz is believed to have witnessed the landing of syphilis in Europe.[2] Haggard records that Diaz wrote a book on the subject dedicated to John III, King of Portugal, which is headed: *Treatise Entitled, Fruit of All Saints Against the Disease of the Island of Espanola . . . to the Common and General Good of those Suffering from the Disease in Question: Commonly Called Bubas . . . .* Diaz had treated syphilis in several of the sailors of Columbus; among these was the pilot, Pinzon, of Palos.

Gabriel Fallopius, the anatomist, after wandering all over Europe 'in order to discover the hidden Secrets of Nature', a practice very common with the medieval physicians as it had been also with those of Greece, wrote in regard to the origin of syphilis:

> Amongst the Genoese was Christopher Columbus, a Man of remarkable Genius, who is called Colonus by Peter Martyr, a careful Writer concerning the Indies. . . . For this Columbus, Ferdinand and Isabella ordered a Frigate to be fitted out, and three Pinnances . . . with which he arrived at the West Indies . . . . There was found there, 'tis true, most precious Gold, and great Plenty of it was brought from thence, together with Aboundance of Pearls; but there was also a thorn joined to the Rose, and Aloes mixed with the Honey. For Columbus brought back his Vessels laden with the French Disease. There the disease is mild like the Itch amongst us, but transplanted hither it is become so fierce and unmerciful, as to infect and corrupt the Head, Eyes, Nose, Palate, Skin, Flesh, Bones, Ligaments, and at last the whole Bowels.[3]

The historian (Haggard) adds:

> It appeared in France, Germany, Switzerland, Holland and Greece in 1496, in Scotland in 1497, and in Hungary and Russia in 1499. The spread of syphilis to the remaining parts of the known world was effected by the great voyagers of the fifteenth and sixteenth centuries. Vasco da Gama carried it on his ships to India in 1498, Europeans brought it to China in 1505, and by 1569 it had been smuggled into Japan. The Jews and Mohamme-dans, who were driven out of Spain by Ferdinand and Isabella after the conquest of Granada, carried the disease to Africa. There is no similar record of such a sudden establishment of any other disease throughout the world. Since the fifteenth century,

this gift of the down-trodden natives of Espanola has been the constant companion of civilized man.

Some recent investigators reject the view that syphilis first evolved among the American Indians, and maintain that a mutation which made it virulent occurred somewhere around the Mediterranean. The exact bacteriological history matters little, as there is general agreement that the disease became virulent in the fifteenth century: its impact on the European mind therefore must date from that time.

It seems unlikely that the physician who treated the sailors of Columbus either made up the story or was completely mistaken about the newness of the disease. On the other hand, the archaeologists have recently found bones from the Roman period which appear to be affected by syphilis. The most plausible conclusion is that the Old World knew a mild type of syphilis and a much more potent strain was brought from America, to which the population of Europe had no resistance.

The sources amply convey the horror which it inspired. Its transmission through copulation was suspected from the beginning, and as it was in fact mostly contracted through unlawful intercourse, it could (more convincingly than any other disease) be regarded as a punishment for that sin. With a little bit of bad luck, one sinful act by either spouse could cause both of them to rot alive, become paralysed or mad, and their offspring be born diseased or dead. Until the nineteenth century the disease was absolutely incurable. A reliable and painless treatment became available only after the discovery of penicillin, which (together with the reliable methods of contraception) made possible the permissive society of today.

In the seventeenth century, mercury began to be used to alleviate some of the effects of syphilis, but this treatment (as we shall see in greater detail in the next chapter) caused poisoning which was often just as bad as the disease.

The Europeans [Haggard says], faced with a new disease, were hard pressed for a name. Each country blamed some other and named the disease accordingly. The Spaniards called it the disease of Espanola; the Italians called it the French disease; the French called it the Italian disease; the English credited it to the French; the Russians named it the Polish disease; for the Turks it was the French disease; and for the Indians and Japanese the Portuguese disease.

It soon became so common that it appeared to Shakespeare as something inevitable. In *Henry IV*, Part 2, Falstaff says:

> A man can no more separate age and covetousness than he can part young limbs and lechery. But the gout galls the one and the pox pinches the other . . . . A pox of this gout! Or a gout of this pox! For the one or the other plays the rogue with my great toe.

Unlike a number of other diseases, which struck more commonly the undernourished, badly housed, and ill clad, syphilis in no way spared the great, and was therefore particularly suited to be viewed as due to God's wrath. It would have been surprising, if seeing such dire consequences of sexual indulgence, people did not begin to view it with horror. Owing to the workings of the well known mental process of generalisation and extension, the abomination of sexual laxity tended to prompt condemnation not only of sexual indulgence within marriage, but also of all other kinds of pleasure or merriment. In other words, on general psychological grounds, the connection between the arrival of syphilis and the wave of asceticism appears very natural.

In an interesting article ('Civilisatie, Besmettingsangst en Hygiene', *Sociologisch Tijdschrift*, Dec. 1977) Johan Goudblom considers the question of whether the awareness and fear of contagion has contributed to the development of hygiene. The evidence confirms the accepted view that until towards the end of the nineteenth century people were totally ignorant about how diseases were transmitted. In view of this ignorance it seems plausible that (as he claims) the fear of disease contributed little to the progress of hygiene until the nineteenth century. None the less, his material shows beyond any doubt that people knew about contagion although they had wrong ideas of how it worked. Here is what Erasmus of Rotterdam makes one of his characters say in a dialogue in *Colloquia* (1523):

> Nothing appears to me more dangerous as that so many people breathe the same warm air . . . there are many who suffer from hidden diseases, and there is no disease which is not contagious.

Surely, many have the Spanish or (as it is often called) French pox, although it appears among all nations. These people present a threat which in my opinion is not smaller than that from the lepers.

The passage comes from Erasmus' colloquy on 'Inns' (1523); six years later he devoted an entire colloquy to the dangers of venereal disease ('A Marriage in Name Only'); there are numerous other passages elsewhere (cf. in the preface of his *Lingue*, 1525 lamenting the ravages of syphilis). Fracastoro's popular Latin poem, *Syphilis* (1530), gave the most epidemic form of the pox (Spanish, Neapolitan, French) its name.

According to Craig Thompson, the editor of a recent edition of Erasmus' *Colloquies* (University of Chicago Press, 1965), the subject was widely treated by both medical and lay contemporaries. Ulrich von Hutten wrote about it (from first-hand experience) in *De morbo Gallico* (1519). Colet exhorted men to 'call to remembrance the marvellous and horrible punishment of the abominable great pox, daily appearing to our sights . . .'. Fisher (in a 1509 sermon) paints a dark picture of men 'vexed with the French pox, poor and needy, lying by the highways stinking and almost rotten above the ground, having intolerable ache in their bones'. One of the charges against Cardinal Wolsey, as Tyndale noted, was that he 'breathed . . . in the king's face when he [Wolsey] had the French pox.'

Although Thompson emphasises that 'its sexual origin was not yet sufficiently understood', Erasmus often associated it with 'intemperate sexuality', when 'young men go whoring', and when women make themselves 'a public sewer that every Tom, Dick, and Harry – the dirty, the vile, the diseased – resorts and empties his filth into . . .' ('The Young Man and the Harlot', 1523, p. 156). Contacts (from 'kissing' to 'common drinking cups') were to be avoided. And Erasmus' friend, Sir Thomas More, even offered a 'Utopian' solution when he tells us that in Utopia an affianced pair are shown to each other naked to prevent ignorance or deception about the health of the future partner.

The Scots seemed to have recognised the venereal character of the disease at an early date; in 1497 the town council of Aberdeen ordered that: 'For protection from the disease which has come out

of France and strange parts, all light women desist from their vice
and sin of venery and work for their support, on pain, else, of
being branded with a hot iron on their cheek and banished from
the town.'

In his edict of 1495 the Emperor Maximilian declared syphilis to
be God's punishment for the sins of men. This remained the
general view throughout the Christian world until recent times,
and was shared, for example, by a physician at the court of Louis
XV who wrote:

> That the Venereal Disease was sent into the World by the
> Disposition of Providence, either to restrain, as with a Bridle,
> the unruly Passions of a sensual Appetite, or as a Scourge to
> correct the Gratification of them, is an Opinion highly probable
> . . . But we must not conclude from hence, that this Disease in
> the Form it now appears, has been therefore known to Ancients,
> because the Lewdness of Mankind has always stood in need of
> a present Correction . . . let us enquire, not what God should
> have done, but what he has done; not whether he ought at all
> Times to have inflicted the Venereal Disease as a Punishment
> for the Lewdness of Mankind; but whether he has in reality so
> punished him or not.[4]

It is equally possible that the advent of the early Christian
asceticism – and the victory of Christianity over the sexually more
permissive religions of Antiquity – might have been connected
with an increase in the virulence of gonorrhoea, which might have
been caused by an increase in mobility and urbanisation produced
by the unification of the Mediterranean world by the Romans.
However, let us leave this hypothesis for the attention of the
specialists able to examine the primary sources and to ascertain
whether in this case there has been a chronological coincidence of
the kind that undoubtedly occurred between syphilis and puritanism in early modern Europe.

The abolition of the celibacy of the clergy can also be regarded as
a move towards greater puritanism ('greater' in the sense of the
more effective and sustained as opposed to more flamboyant but
commonly contravened) because it brought the commandments of

religion within the bounds of practicability. Although most people find strict marital fidelity difficult enough, there had been times and societies where many – perhaps a considerable majority – did maintain it; and, provided the age of marriage was not very high, also observed premarital chastity. In contrast only a few exceptional individuals can observe life-long chastity. Consequently, despite being designed to exclude temptation, even monasteries and nunneries often had the reputation (probably at least partially deserved) of being hotbeds of secret fornication and buggery, while infringements of celibacy have always been common among the lay clergy. Faced with impossibly high demands, the Catholic clergy have never been able to abide so steadfastly by the rules of their calling as did their Protestant equivalents who, even in the most puritanical denominations, had a much easier task, as they were allowed to marry.

Until the general weakening of the influence of religion which has occurred during the present century, consistent observance of the acknowledged rules of sexual morality was more common among the Protestants than among the Catholics who could obtain absolution through confession, while the former (with the partial exception of the Church of England) had no such escape from guilt and damnation. Another broad difference between the two religions lies in the unequal weight assigned to the sins of men and women, in which respect the Protestants approached equality more closely, whereas the Catholics (with the exception of the Irish) have treated men's sexual misdemeanours much less seriously. This contrast may, however, stem from other circumstances (including pre-Christian traditions), since most Catholics live in countries stamped by the Mediterreanean culture whereas most Protestants are Nordics, among whom women had a higher status even in prehistoric times. It may be, therefore, that on this point it was the religion that was moulded by the regional traditions rather than the other way round; or, as so often happens, the influence was reciprocal. However this may have been, the diminution of the concessions made to men can be interpreted as an adaptation to the epidemic of syphilis.

The increased strictness of the Catholic Church during the Counter-Reformation is usually explained as a reaction to the danger of disintegration and a result of the wars of religion. That greater intolerance of dissent might thus have been evoked seems highly likely, but the link between this and the tightening up of sexual morality seems tenuous. It seems more likely that the Catholic Church was affected by the factor, operating throughout Europe, which was also steering the development of the Protestant ethics in the direction of sexual puritanism. Anyway, there is no need to insist on monocausality and regard these explanations as mutually exclusive, as the impact of syphilis could have been reinforced by the effects of the struggle.

My thesis linking the rise of Puritanism (as well as the diffusion of puritanism) with the spread of syphilis finds further support from the absence of convincing alternative explanations. There is no reason to assume that the clusters of beliefs and commandments which crystallised as the doctrines of the denominations known to history were predetermined; and that no other combinations could have succeeded in establishing themselves, if some of the circumstances had been different. In comparison with the policy of the medieval Church, Calvin widened economic freedom while narrowing sexual freedom – not so much by introducing new restrictions as by a much stricter enforcement of the old prohibitions of fornication and adultery. Now, no compensating mechanism has been discovered whereby the lifting of the ban on usury and large profits would entail a greater severity towards the sins of the flesh, or the other way round. The existing explanations of this cluster of tenets invoke the notions and idiosyncrasies of the founder, which leaves it unexplained why the 'package' offered by him was absorbed by large multitudes while the packages offered by other prophets fell on deaf ears. As a matter of fact, the first wave of the Reformation (inaugurated by Martin Luther) seems to have been accompanied by a relaxation of sexual restrictions which reached its most extreme form in the marital communism of Thomas Müntzer. The trend towards puritanism was led by John Calvin, but it seems implausible to attribute it entirely to his powers of persuasion.

In his *Peasant War in Germany* Friedrich Engels explains Calvinism as the religion of the merchant based on idolisation of parsimony. This interpretation of Calvinism as an adaptation to the needs of developing capitalism seems plausible in so far as it concerns the tenets which affect the conduct of business. The prohibition of lending on interest, the condemnation of high profits and accumulation of capital, the ethical regulation of conditions of employment and the obligations of charity and heavy donations to the Church did impede the development of capitalism; and their removal must have facilitated this process. Furthermore, it seems likely that businessmen would be inclined to support a doctrine which not only freed them from irksome restrictions but also bestowed a blessing on occupational inclinations which the medieval Church damned as sinful greed.

In contrast, there is no evidence that mercantile activity as such fosters an abhorrence of carnal pleasures. In Tokugawa Japan and Sung China the merchants were criticised by scholars for their inclination to sybaritism (the word comes, significantly, from the name of a commercial city in ancient Greece). The Italian merchants – Europe's first capitalists – were not known to be averse to the pleasures of bed or table. In most times and places the extent of hedonism depended on the means, while the 'inner-wordly asceticism' in the midst of wealth appears as something extraordinary in the light of comparative history. From the psychological viewpoint, therefore, the link between commerce and asceticism appears extraneous or accidental – that is, produced by circumstances external to both. The causation normally works in the opposite direction: frugality helps in making money which (at least in the following generations) prompts self-indulgence, which in turn puts an end to the acquisition of wealth – at least through productive work. In contrast, the mental processes through which an epidemic of syphilis might have elicited puritanism and inner-wordly asceticism appear as psychologically understandable and, indeed, 'natural.'

We must not, however, push the thesis to the point of one-sidedness. It seems unlikely that the linking of the abhorrence of pleasure with the dedication to work would have occurred without other circumstances which distinguished North-Western Europe (and later, to an even greater extent, New England) from the rest of the world: such as the fairly ample opportunities to reap the fruits of one's labour, connected with the considerable freedoms and status of the merchants, craftsmen, and to a lesser extent even peasants. In different times and other places the puritan inclinations led more often to unproductive self-mortification than to enterprise or to invention. The Russian 'Skoptzy', for example, found an outlet for their puritanism in the custom of undergoing castration.

Max Weber was right in thinking that the greatest originality of the puritanical variants of Protestantism was the 'inner-wordly asceticism' which prompted unremitting work and abstemiousness, regardless of financial success. Such ethics could seldom fail to stimulate the accumulation of capital and (what was at least equally crucial) its investment in productive equipment rather than in appurtenances of ostentatious consumption and in self-indulgence. It stands to reason that lineages maintaining these attitudes over the generations would be better at building up family firms than people of less austere frame of mind, and more likely to get to the top in economic competition. It would be strange if countries with many persons of this kind would not develop faster along capitalistic lines than countries where they were few. What Max Weber did not, of course, say is that a *medical* factor might have been involved in the causation of this superiority.

In the absence of statistical data we can only surmise – but it seems likely that, given the virulence and incurability of syphilis, a stricter observance of marital fidelity and premarital chastity would bestow upon a family, a lineage, a region, a country, or a population demarcated by religion, a considerable advantage in health and in vigour. This factor might have played a part in the more rapid progress of the Protestant countries, as well as in the economic ascendancy of Protestant minorities in Catholic regions or nations. The 'medical factor' would thus reinforce the effects of cultural traits.

The debate which arose around Max Weber's thesis has given birth to a vast literature which could not be considered here, no matter how summarily, without doubling the length of the present chapter. (In any case I have presented my view on this matter in an article incorporated in an expanded form in the book *Max Weber's Insights and Errors.*)[5] My conclusion is that, provided that we do not think in simplistic terms of single and one-way causation, and admit reciprocal influence, Weber was right in maintaining that puritanism helped the growth of capitalism.

It seems likely – or at least conceivable – that without this stimulus the forces tending to arrest this development might have triumphed. The case of the Low Countries supports this view: until the Reformation the chief centres of business enterprise in Northern Europe were located in what is now Belgian territory, the most prominent being Bruges and Antwerp. Later these centres stagnated or withered under the rule of the Habsburgs and the

Catholic Church, while Protestant Holland began to lead the world not only in commerce but in science, technology, and agriculture as well. Cross-Channel learning from the Dutch underlay the commercial and technical advances of England. It seems likely that this chain of developments would have been broken had the Spaniards been able to subdue the Netherlands and extirpate the Dutch Reformed Church.

I have tried to show that the impact of syphilis played a crucial role in the formation of puritanism as well as in the 'puritanisation' of the Catholic Church. The influence on the Lutheran and the Anglican Churches must have been similar.

One could also look at puritanism as an adaptive reaction which permitted the preservation of healthy genetic lines and the growth of population despite the disease. People of stern morals, who avoided fornication and adultery and who chose as spouses persons of similar conduct, had a much better chance of a long life and of producing a large and healthy progeny, whereas libertines died young and left a few sickly descendants. Owing to the pressure of the population upon resources, and the high death rate among the physically or financially weak – aggravated below the upper classes by a vicious circle of poverty and debility – the lines contaminated by syphilis were constantly eliminated and replaced by the offspring of families with stern sexual morals. Thus, there was a biological selection for puritanism. As morals among the upper classes were laxer than among the lower, the degeneration and dying out of noble families must have fostered an upward social mobility which facilitated Europe's cultural innovation.

Neither science and technology nor the other extraordinary traits of Western civilisation could have developed without capitalism. And now it seems that among the circumstances which helped its rise a dark 'medical factor' – syphilis – played an important role. Such are the surprising mysteries of social causation.

The medical factor also throws a new light on a feature of Calvinism which is out of harmony with its ethic of striving and hard work: namely, the belief in predestination. Owing to the unawareness of the connection between them, no explanation of the adoption of this belief has been offered, leaving aside simple attributions of this mass phenomenon to Calvin's personal idiosyncrasy. As far as the effects are concerned, most scholars repeat Max Weber's view that this belief acted as a spur to work and enterprise because people were eager to find out as quickly as possible whether they were among the chosen or the damned. Psychologically, however, this seems very implausible: why should you strive if it can make no difference because the outcome is pre-ordained? Since you can do nothing about it, why not relax or do whatever tickles your fancy? Belief in predestination is much more likely to foster passivity and resignation than a spirit of enterprise. Indeed, the decline or stagnation of the Oriental lands is often attributed to the attitudes engendered by this belief, which is called fatalism in this context. Why should the same idea have opposite effects in the West and in the East?

The explanation of this incongruity is that the Calvinists never took to heart their founder's tenet about predestination, and profoundly believed that one's destiny is in one's own hands. All the material adduced by Weber reveals an activist attitude to life. There is nothing unusual about such selectivity of which there are many examples in all religions and doctrines. For example: after the early communes, the Christians took no notice of Jesus's counsel to offer the other cheek and brandished crosses in the midst of murderous battles. The Oriental fatalism has deep roots in the way of life: it is an adaptation to living at the mercy of cruel despots on whose whimsical commands one's fate depends much more than on one's merit or effort. For women listlessness and resignation are an inevitable adaptation to being treated as chattels without will or mind of their own. The attitude of the mother is inevitably imbibed not only by the daughters but also by the sons. This fatalism stems from the conditions of life rather than directly from the statements in the Koran which encourage it.

Calvin's pronouncements about predestination were treated by his followers as a purely theoretical point of no greater practical significance than Christ's condemnation of wealth in the parable about the camel and the eye of the needle. Neither deterred them from working like beavers and saving like squirrels. The superficially held predestinarian dogma played only a minor role in stimulating the accumulation of capital by serving as an excuse for abandoning the old Christian commandment of charity: for, if people were poor because they were damned by God, then they deserved no alms.

The decline of charity in the early period of Puritanism stimulated the development of capitalism firstly because, being unable to count upon being rescued by others, people had a greater incentive to accumulate capital as an insurance against ill luck. Secondly, for the poor it became even more difficult to survive without working. Consequently, they would view laziness in a child with horror, as it was a sure road to an early grave.

Industriouness and accumulation necessarily followed from the abhorrence of pleasures coupled with the rejection of passive asceticism. This rejection was partly due to the role of the monastic orders as the Pope's army whom the Protestants were obliged to fight; and partly to the natural hostility of busy craftsmen and traders to parasitic monks. Given that contemplative self-mortification and dedication to a joyless activity are alternative ways of avoiding pleasure, a rejection of one leaves only the other, as sheer idleness can plausibly be viewed as self-indulgent and conducive to sin.

Whereas the rejection of the monastic alternative can thus be regarded as due to socio-political circumstances, the abhorrence of pleasures stemmed (as we saw earlier) from a generalisation of the well-grounded fear of the consequences of indulgence. But whence did the notion of predestination come? It was contrary not only to the ethic of work but also to all the ideas about the wages of sin and the rewards of purity. No light upon this mystery can be found in an economic interpretation which sees in Puritanism an emanation of the outlook of businessmen who can hardly be suspected of having a natural bent towards fatalism. To find a more convincing solution we must look again at the impact of syphilis: the idea of predestination acquired a particular plausibility when more often than ever people could see innocent children suffering for the sins of their fathers and mothers.

According to Reed's *Textbook of the Practice of Medicine*:[6]

An infected mother can transmit syphilis to her offspring long after she has ceased to be sexually contagious. In general the more recent her infection the more severe the effects of transmitted infection on the foetus. The theoretical course of the obstetric history of a syphilitic woman is stated in Kassowitz's Law, according to which each pregnancy results in miscarriage progressively later in pregnancy, followed by the delivery of stillborn or macerated fetuses at term, then by living syphilitic infants and finally by healthy infants. This kind of history, which is presumed to be due to gradual attenuation of infection, is

seldom obtained. In practice, miscarriage may alternate with
stillborn or living syphilitic children and a healthy infant may
be born between two who are infected. It has even occurred that
only one of twins was syphilitic.

Aggravated by the element of unpredictability, the lack of
understanding of the causation was one of the reasons (as we shall
see later) why the crop of congenital diseases, malformations and
still births fanned the fear of and the hunts for witches. In many
cases, however, the link with the sins of the progenitors was so
obvious that it could be understood even in the light of the
rudimentary medical knowledge of the times. The sight of afflic-
tions, which in no way could be treated as a retribution for
the sufferer's sins, provoked much discussion of how this was
compatible with God's justice. The idea of predestination, which
received from the circumstances an increment of plausibility,
presented a way of dodging the issue.

The impact of the epidemic of syphilis on culture was thus
double-edged at two junctures: the abhorrence of pleasures, which
it engendered, could stimulate either dedication to work or contemplative self-mortification. Among the Catholics it seems to have
done both, but among the Protestants the second outcome was
barred by the political and economic circumstances: so, only the
former remained. Secondly, the dogma of predestination, fostered
by the disease, might have induced fatalism, had the circumstances
been conducive to an attitude of resignation, but the economic and
political situation of the main bearers of Calvinism prompted them
to treat it as a purely theoretical point and to draw no practical
lessons from it other than an excuse for a refusal of charity.

Although other factors also played crucial roles in fostering the
extraordinary intellectual and economic progress of north-western
Europe since the Reformation, its occurrence fits very well Freud's
theory. Albeit usually presented as the prophet of permissiveness,
Freud believed that civilisation was the product of sublimation of
the sexual desire. Repression from the field of consciousness of
erotic impulses and fantasies by the emotions of guilt and shame
('the censor') could, according to him, direct the energy of the
libido either through the channel of 'regression' into the production
of neuroses, or through the channel of 'sublimation' into an activity
dedicated to a non-hedonistic goal, that is not guided by the search
for pleasure. For example, the non-utilitarian curiosity, which

created science, stems, in Freud's view, from frustrated sexual curiosity. It follows from this theory that an injection of puritanism into a culture might have two different (in a way opposite) kinds of effects: on the one hand, it ought to stimulate purposeful activities whether of a constructive kind (such as inventiveness and business enterprise) or of an aggressive kind like conquests and revolutions. On the other, it should foster private as well as collective neuroses such as religious or doctrinaire manias. This is what did in fact occur in Europe after the epidemic of syphilis had struck: unprecedented intellectual and technical progress on one side; religious fanaticism, persecutions and manias on the other.

Although Freud's scheme points to a factor of crucial importance, it cannot alone provide an adequate explanation of the rise of science and business enterprise which needed other favourable circumstances: where these were absent (as in Spain and Russia) the additional energies generated by greater sexual inhibitions appear to have found outlets only in religious fanaticism, persecutions and fighting which among the progressive nations constituted only one side of the picture. However, one of the crazes (not the most destructive but the nearest to insanity) caused much greater ravages in the progressive north-western Europe than on its stagnant southern and eastern peripheries: this was the persecutory obsession with witches. This craze calls for a special attention because it was connected with the epidemic of syphilis not only through the effects of puritanism (in the general non-denominational sense) but also by more direct causal links. However, before we turn to this extraordinary phenomenon let me draw your attention to another inference from the psychoanalytic theory.

If Freud is right, the advent of sexual permissiveness (made possible by contraceptives and penicillin) ought to act as a sedative, dampening the creative energies as well as the aggressive impulses and manias. This seems to be in fact the case, although affluence and the consequent absence of physical suffering constitutes another factor to which the increased placidity of the Europeans and the North Americans can be attributed. An opportunity to assess the separate effects of the sexual factor alone would arise if a retreat from permissiveness and a revival of puritanism took place without a collapse of the affluence, as could happen if the population were struck by a powerful and incurable new venereal disease.

Note: The preceding paragraph was written before the appearance of Aids, the possible social consequences of which are discussed in Appendix One.

Notes

1. William McNeill, *Players and Peoples* (Oxford: Basil Blackwell, 1977).
2. Howard H. Haggard, *Devils, Drugs and Doctors* (Springfield, Ill.: C. C. Thomas, 1959) pp. 249–50.
3. Ibid.
4. Quoted by Haggard, p. 160.
5. Stanislav Andreski, *Max Weber's Insights and Errors* (London: Routledge and Kegan Paul, 1982).
6. Price, *Textbook of the Practice of Medicine*, 12th edn, ed. Sir Ronald Badley Scott (Oxford University Press, 1978) p. 105.

2

Syphilis, Celibacy and Witch Hunts

The Witch Hunts of the sixteenth and seventeenth centuries present one of the most bizarre and gruesome spectacles to be found in the history of mankind. My interest was drawn to this extraordinary phenomenon in connection with a critique of Max Weber's concept of rationalisation which can be shown as misleading on various other grounds as well, but which the evidence of the Witch Hunts suffices to discredit.[1] For how can we speak of the European outlook or the Western way of life becoming more 'rational' or 'rationalised' during the era when people were in the grip of a mania which fits better the label of irrationality than any other form of mass behaviour recorded by history?

Unless we want to make it synonymous with the lack of knowledge or with error (and therefore superfluous as a concept) we must define irrationality as an attitude to knowledge, character-ised by the inclination to hold on to a belief or to persist in the choice of a means to a given end, despite the availability of the knowledge which shows it to be erroneous. With this definition, we cannot say that the Dobu Islanders' beliefs about witchcraft were irrational since, given their knowledge, they had no good reasons for regarding them as false. In contrast, we can assert that the striking spread of preoccupation with witchcraft in Europe after 1500, which continued for more than a century, did constitute a growth of irrationality because it occurred despite the accumu-lation of knowledge. We cannot explain Isaac Newton's or Robert Boyle's credulity by supposing that they did not know enough to appreciate the reasons which led Francis Bacon or Michel de Montaigne to incredulity a century earlier. The eagerness to silence the critics by censorship and persecution suggests that the theoreticians of Witch Hunts did not feel completely secure in their beliefs. As is well known, anyone who criticised the beliefs or procedures was accused of being in league with devils and witches, and therefore a witch him- or herself.

21

There are many gripping and exhaustive accounts of the facts but the explanations are few, and even the most ingenious of them seem to me inadequate – at least in the sense that although they may explain a particular feature within a given region, they fail to account for the generality of the phenomenon. However, might we not suppose that there is no need for a general explanation because the same kind of behaviour was prompted by different circumstances in each region? I don't see how one could refute conclusively such an interpretation; but it seems very improbable that a clustering of such activities could be due to sheer coincidence. However, perhaps we could be satisfied with regarding it simply as a wave of imitation, with the added (and well-founded) assumption that absurdity does not preclude imitation.

This point raises great difficulties. The propensity to imitate undoubtedly constitutes one of the most fundamental character-istics of our species, ineradicably rooted in its social nature. For any single individual, this propensity provides a sufficient explanation of why he or she resembles in so many ways those among whom he or she lives. On the collective level, moreover, there is something which might be called the momentum of a wave of imitation. Once a pattern of behaviour has been widely initiated, it acquires a self-perpetuating force which is (at least partly) independent of the circumstances which promoted it initially. This factor must be taken into account despite our inability to assess its weight within a degree of approximation which is better than very rough. However, the propensity to imitate – which is universal and probably constant among large populations – cannot explain why in a given time and place a certain pattern is imitated rather than another. We must, therefore, search for factors which might have predisposed people to imitate what they did. Our explanation, moreover, must be in terms of phenomena of the same order of generality as the explanandum.

I wish to make clear that I am offering no explanation of why people believe in magic or in witchcraft, which is a special form of it. I merely note that in all pre-scientific cultures people think that you can harm or help other persons (or yourself, for that matter) by pronouncing certain words ('incantations') or performing certain acts ('rituals'). Many illustrious thinkers – from Herbert Spencer and Edward Taylor to Emile Durkheim and Bronislaw Malinowski – have addressed themselves to the task of explaining the universality of such beliefs, and I have nothing new to add on this question.

My sole purpose here is to explain the change which occurred in Europe during the sixteenth and seventeenth centuries: the striking intensification of the fear of witchcraft. The belief that it worked was the underlying condition which permitted the Great Witch Craze to occur but it cannot account for its flaring up, because a constant cannot account for a change. Another factor must have acted as a precipitant.

There is a consensus among historians that the Witch Craze was not a continuation of the tradition but something unprecedented in its intensity which was connected with a striking change in the attitude of the Church. According to Hugh Trevor-Roper:

> In the eighth century, we find St Boniface, the English apostle of Germany, declaring roundly that to believe in witches and werewolves is unchristian. In the same century Charlemagne decreed the death penalty for anyone who, in newly converted Saxony, burnt supposed witches. Such burning, he said, was 'a pagan custom.' In the next century, St Agobard, Bishop of Lyon, repudiated the belief that witches could make bad weather and another unknown Church dignitary declared that night-flying and metamorphosis were hallucinations and that whoever believed in them 'is beyond doubt an infidel and a pagan.' This statement was accepted into the canon law and became known as the *canon Episcopi* or *capitulum Episcopi*. It remained the official doctrine of the Church. In the eleventh century the laws of King Coloman of Hungary declined to notice witches 'since they do not exist', and the twelfth-century John of Salisbury dismissed the idea of a witches' sabbat as a fabulous dream. In the succeeding centuries, when the craze was being built up, all this salutary doctrine would have to be reversed. The laws of Charlemagne and Coloman would be forgotten; to deny the reality of night-flying and metamorphosis would be officially declared heretical; the witches' sabbat would become an objective fact, disbelieved only (as a doctor of the Sorbonne would write in 1609) by those of unsound mind; and the ingenuity of churchmen and lawyers would be taxed to explain away that inconvenient text of canon law, the *canon Episcopi* . . .[2]

The oldest explanation – which goes back to the wonderfully brave eye-witness critics of this practice – attributes it to ignorance and stupidity. No doubt the general ignorance of the population still uninfluenced by the discoveries of science constituted a general underlying condition; but we have no evidence that ignorance or stupidity increased in other fields of culture. So we would have a perfectly circular explanation if we took the persecution of witches as evidence of the state of mind to which this practice is attributed.

Like many people after them, the eighteenth century philosophers regarded Witch Trials as a relic of the barbarian past to which the Enlightenment based on science had put an end. Their view of why these trials ceased is perfectly tenable because it is true that this occurred at the time when the discoveries of science began to influence the outlook of all educated persons. However, because historical research was only in its very beginnings, these thinkers did not know that the two centuries which preceded theirs did not represent a fair picture of the earlier times, and that never before had the Europeans been so obsessed with this particular superstition as during the two centuries which witnessed the birth of science and revival of scholarship and philosophy. The great intensification of the persecutions at such a time demands a specific explanation which cannot be in terms of sheer inertia of tradition. On the other hand, the common acceptance of the belief in witchcraft was an underlying and pre-existing condition without which the said intensification could not have occurred, and which can be attributed to cultural inertia and some very widely spread mental tendencies. However, inertia of old beliefs may have accounted up to a point for the behaviour of peasants but not for the well-documented change in the attitude of the intellectuals who abandoned the limited scepticism of their predecessors, became just as (if not more) obsessed with the fear of witches as the peasants, and played a crucial role in inciting and organising the hunts.

EXPLANATIONS

Let me begin a brief survey of the explanations of the great Witch Hunt with the latest, which also happens to be the flimsiest.

In her book, *Die Hexen der Neuzeit*[4] Claudia Honegger interprets the Witch Trials as a part of the process (if not a deliberate method) of lowering women's status and bolstering up patriarchy. Although not all historians would agree with her assessment of the trend, let us assume that she is right in what she says about the changes in 'the position of women.' Even if we admitted that the wave of Witch Trials did contribute to a lowering of this position, it would not follow that one would have discovered their hidden purpose. Such a conclusion would be warranted only if we had grounds for believing that Witch Trials were motivated (if not entirely, then at least to a large extent) by the desire to subjugate the female population.

The first reason for rejecting such a surmisal is that too many men and boys were burnt. It is true – and it is a fact which I shall endeavour to explain – that at the beginning of the sixteenth century, not only did the number of the victims drastically increase, but also the sex ratio among them changed to women's disadvantage. None the less, in absolute numbers the number of male victims also seems to have increased, and they constituted (according to the estimates summarised by Jean Delumeau[4]) about one-fourth or one-fifth of the total number. Even if it is true (as some historians maintain) that males constituted only 10% or 15% of the victims, it is scarcely conceivable that so many men would have been burnt if the aim were to frighten women into submission.

An equally strong argument against viewing witch-burning as a strategy of 'sex war' is that resorting to it would be as rational as using a sledge-hammer to crack a nut: it is better to have a slave than a corpse, and there is no need for torture and burning when simple beating would be enough for the purpose. The Moslems have always maintained women in much greater subjection without recourse to the methods of the witch-hunters. In our own days, Khomeini and his faithful have been able to roll back in Iran the worldwide tide of women's emancipation and to put them back into a very inferior position with the aid of intimidation backed up by a few stonings.

More ingenious is the explanation put forth by Keith Thomas.[5] As is fashionable nowadays, Thomas turns to the economic factors but he adds an interesting application of some psychological or psychoanalytic concepts. The influence of capitalism upon rural life, according to his thesis, led to the destruction of village solidarity and a clash between the duty to help the unfortunate neighbours and the pursuit of self-enrichment. People who were growing rich no longer complied with this duty, but the tradition was still strong enough to make them feel guilty about keeping all their wealth for themselves. Now, according to the psychoanalysts, when feelings of guilt are repressed from the consciousness, they tend to be 'projected' on to those who have been wronged. The wrongdoer denies that he has wronged them, and not only imputes to the wronged hostile feelings towards him, but also convinces himself that they are actively doing or have done something to harm him. Refusing help to poor old women would be especially likely to make the budding capitalists feel guilty, and therefore poor old women would be the most common objects of a 'projection' which would then prompt suspicions and accusations. Thomas backs his thesis by an examination of the materials from the English courts, where he finds that a victim of accusation has often been previously refused aid.

Although it is quite possible that situations of this kind did on some occasions trigger off a victimisation, as a general explanation Thomas's thesis seems inadequate despite its ingenuity. Firstly, on psychological grounds. A 'projection' of guilt could have prompted avoidance or further harassment of the wronged without going to such extremes. It could also have led to an espousal of a belief which justified the refusal to help and removed the feelings of guilt. Indeed, the link between John Calvin's doctrine of predestination and the development of capitalism probably rested on its appeal as a justification for leaving the poor to their fate, on the grounds that they are poor because they have been damned by God. Perhaps quite often the process of 'repressing' and 'projecting' such guilt feelings might have determined who was picked up for victimisation once the hunt was on; but it is difficult to imagine how it could have produced the widely shared obsessional fear which constituted the necessary background of these events.

A comparative view yields an even more decisive argument against accepting Keith Thomas's thesis as a general explanation. If the Witch Craze had been a by-product of development of Capitalism, it should have been most virulent where this development started earliest or went furthest – Italy, the Low Countries, and England – but this was not the case. Indeed, though affected, these countries suffered a good deal less than France and Germany where the village community was much less (indeed, hardly at all) disturbed by new capitalist enterprise. Furthermore, in neither of these countries had there been a clustering of the trials around the centres of capitalism – the Hanseatic cities or Paris – while many of the bloodiest persecutions occurred in remote rural areas like the foothills of the Alps or Aquitaine. It appears from the not exactly comparable estimates made by A. Macfarlane and G. F. Black,[6] that about twenty times more witches were burnt in rustic and sparsely inhabited Scotland than in the five counties round London, the population of which was not much smaller. The craze reached Poland late and began to rage only during the seventeenth century when the cities were decaying and the very rudimentary capitalism was in full regression.

The final argument against Keith Thomas's thesis as a general explanation is that what he says about the social positions of the victims he has studied does not seem to apply to other samples. Soldan, Heppe and Bauel[7] give long lists of victims in various places in Germany where we find traders, artisans, squires, priests, burgomasters and even a High Court judge. Only the high nobility are absent. In her study of Luxembourg, Dupont-Bouchat[8] found mayors, magistrates and rich merchants, while E. W. Monter[9] found wives of men of equivalent rank among the victims of the trials in the Jura.

The same argument applies with an even greater force against the view put forth by Jeanne Favret[10] that the Witch Hunts formed a part of (or were a manifestation of) 'class conflict.'

The persecutions, she argues, were instigated not by peasants but by the judges, whose motive was fear of the counter-culture of the weak. This last point is an unwarranted extrapolation of a notion which was perhaps not without applicability to the recent situation in France and a few other countries in 1968 when the 'hippies' were throwing down gauntlets to the 'squares'. Perhaps also the ideas and the way of life of the anarchist and communist groups, which have kept on springing up since the French Revolution, could be regarded as a 'counter-culture' which presented a challenge to the established culture and, therefore, inspired fear in the official circles. As far as the old Europe is concerned, there is no evidence that the folkways of peasants (let alone of the starving vagabonds) were regarded as a danger or a challenge by royalty and the nobility. Nor could the rebellious peasants think of any innovations, and they justified their complaints by traditional references to the Bible. True, the nobility did have reasons to fear the numerical strength of the peasants; but they always took good precautions to keep them under the yoke, and did not need the pretext of witchcraft to mete out atrocious punishments. The sanguinary reprisals against peasant uprisings and banditry claimed many more victims than the Witch Trials: instead of individual burnings, entire fields were covered with impaled rebels. The Witch Hunts, moreover, would have been a very inappropriate method of nipping resistance in the bud because they were biased not against the most dangerous category – young men – but against the least dangerous – single women. True, even lonely and poor old women were evidently regarded as dangerous by powerful and rich men: but the question is *why*?

Nothing one reads in histories of the trials supports the view that their aim was to suppress eccentricity or dissent. If that were the case, there would be no need to resort to elaborate tracking of suspects or to extorting confessions by torture. The justification given by the demonologists for torture was that the witches cannot be detected by obvious characteristics of appearance or behaviour. Most seem to have been very ordinary people who had the misfortune that someone saw a black cat walking in and out or a bat or an owl hovering around the house, or some other trivial event which the superstition endowed with great portent. No doubt eccentricity or mental illness increased the danger of arousing suspicions, but it is very far-fetched to imagine that an assortment of unlucky people constituted a group in any proper meaning of this word, let alone a defiant counter-culture.

Favret is on safer ground when she claims that most of the processes were initiated by the judges or judicial officials. This is confirmed by Baschwitz and Mandrou,[11] and it is hardly surprising since they had the power. On the other hand, there are many examples of popular initiative and lynchings even when the trials were already forbidden by the princes or the parliament as was the case in Poland. The 'Witch-Finder General', Matthew Hopkins, for example, started a business after the Civil War, travelling to various places in England at the request of the local population in the grip of a panic, and receiving payment from them piece-rate. The fact that most of the victims were peasants (57% on Delumeau's reckoning) proves no bias against them since everywhere they constituted at least eight-tenths (if not nine-tenths) of the population. In any case, too many victims were of respectable status to permit an interpretation of the Witch Trials as a method of keeping down the poor.

In his article on witchcraft, Lucien Fèvre thus summarises a case which he regards as typical.[12] It exemplifies no bias either against women or the poor.

Elisabeth became a widow at the age of twenty-four.

She is devout and rather fanatical and thinks she will retire to a convent. One fine day in 1618 a relation of hers persuades her to go on a pilgrimage to Remiremont. When she has finished her devotions she goes and sits down in an inn. There is a doctor there called Charles Poirot. He is struck by Elisabeth's beauty. He fusses around her, courts her and offers her food and drink. At one point during the proceedings, when the doctor has put a piece of salted bacon on her plate, which is a particular delicacy in Lorraine, Elisabeth notices that it is not salted bacon. It is a love philtre which Poirot has given her and from that moment onwards she is under the doctor's spell.

At the same time as she took delight in it she was horrified by it. More precisely (and this is the reason why she was horrified by it) it was not she herself who delighted in it but 'the Other'. One day when she met Poirot she fainted. She felt the doctor 'breathe on her a breath which contained a spell'. Straight away she showed all the signs of severe hysteria of the sort described by Charcot – paralysis of one half of the body, loss of taste, smell, touch and hearing etc. The apothecary was consulted, who sent her to the doctor. That is to say Poirot, who hastened to attend to her. She sent him away. Then called him back. Then she sent him away again. The priest who was informed gave his opinion; it was the Devil. He sent her to Nancy where specialists were to exorcise her.

This was done and Elisabeth remained cured until the day when she met Poirot again. There was a relapse. New exorcisms. Wrong exit by the Devil 'with a terrible noise', and the doctors were called in again; they washed their hands of the affair, it was a matter for the exorcisers. And for six years without a break the exorcisers applied themselves to driving out the Devil.

One day Poirot, who was passing through Nancy, had the

stupid idea of attending a session with Elisabeth. She recognized him and fell into a trance, denouncing him. He was arrested. His case was entrusted to the *élite* of the magistrates of Lorraine. On 30 March 1621 all the hair was shaved off his body and pins were stuck in him until the mark of Satan was discovered. On 24 April he was interrogated. He confessed nothing. But by the end of November a young peasant girl who was suspected of witchcraft had introduced his name into the affair. And the case started anew. They looked for the mark on her and found it. It spelt death for Poirot.

But the doctor had his supporters in France, Italy and Flanders. Philip II's own daughter, the Infanta Isabella-Clara-Eugenie wrote about the case to the Duke of Lorraine. But the twenty-four judges appointed, who were the most truthworthy and the wisest that could be found, unanimously declared Poirot guilty. He was throttled, together with the peasant girl. Their bodies were burned.

Although on the whole soldiers were seldom picked upon, even officers were not entirely beyond the reach of the Witch Hunters. In *The Geography of Witchcraft*, Montague Summers describes the case of a major in Scotland, quoting from the Court proceedings:

the Major did accordinglie confess unto him that he was guilty of Adulterie, Incest, &c., and desired the deponer to pray for him as a persone guiltie of the said grievous crymes; and farder declares, that after the Major was brought down out of the Tolbuith, and the deponer being desired to retier with him to the little roum before the Toune's Councill hous, he did confess again, &c., and the deponer having asked him if he had seen the Deivell, he answered, that any fealling he ever hade of him was in the dark; and this is treuth, &c." The process being thus ended the jury did unanimously find the Major guilty of Incest with his sister, and bestiality with a Mare, and a Cow, and found him guilty of Adultery and Fornication by a plurality of votes. Whereupon the deputed Judges sentenced him to be strangled at a stake betwixt Edinburgh and Leith, on Monday following, the 11th of April, and his body to be burnt to ashes—a sentence executed at the Galla-lee, where, however, it would seem, that this miserable wretch was actually burned alive. This shameful circumstance is thus recorded, "That the body of this unclean Beast gave manifest tokens of its impurity, as soon as it began to be heated by the flames. In the flames along with him was consumed his conjuring staff, carved with heads like those of Satyrs, without which he could not pray, nor work many of his other diabolical feats.[13]

Alan Macfarlane's explanation is also economic but he combines it (in contrast with Keith Thomas) with some ideas brought from anthropology rather than psychoanalysis.[14] He also thinks that the wave of Witch Trials was caused by 'the rise of capitalism' but sees the connection as the opposite of a class conflict. His materials show that the accusations were usually made against neighbours or at least persons with whom the accusers had been in close contact. This means that the Witch Hunts were a grass-roots movement rather than something engineered 'from above', which is the opposite of the picture given by Mandrou.[15] Personally, I doubt whether either of them is wrong about the cases which he examined; it seems to me clear that their materials simply illustrate the variations which did in fact occur.

Macfarlane takes his clue from the studies of Witchcraft in contemporary Africa where the anthropologists have noticed that (contrary to what might be expected *a priori*) townsmen, who appear to be modernised, engage in witchcraft more readily than people who have remained in tribal villages hardly touched by the science-based civilisation. This paradox was first reported by Monica Hunter-Wilson in 1935, in her book, *Reaction to Conquest*. Her explanation was that witchcraft is more tempting when additional curbs are put on physical violence, while everyday conflicts become more intractable owing to the absence or irrelevance of regulation by deeply-rooted customs. Many later studies have corroborated this view. Macfarlane applies this interpretation to the England of the seventeenth century and maintains that the penetration of monetary economy into the villages disclocated the traditional structure, bred more frequent and intense conflicts, and thereby stimulated witchcraft.

The first objection against Macfarlane's thesis is the same as against Keith Thomas':[5] namely, that a comparative survey reveals little (if not an inverse) connection between the development of capitalism and the dimensions of the persecutions, as many of the most sanguinary hunts took place in rural areas unaffected by commerce or industry. The second weakness of the thesis is the assumption that an increase in the number of trials indicates more frequent recourse to witchcraft. We may believe the anthropologists who tell us that they have observed such an increase in Africa. About the seventeenth century we have no statements from independent observers, trained in objectivity and free to report. Confessions wrung out by torture tell us nothing except what the tormentors wanted to hear. Nor does the number of accusations prove anything about the frequency of the practice. For how can I know that someone is bewitching me in secret unless their incantations and rites do in fact produce the desired effect? On the other hand, if people are in the habit of attributing their ills to witchcraft, then any increase in misfortunes will prompt an increase in the number of accusations.

Nor can we presume that there is a close connection between intensity of conflicts and frequency of accusations, unless we have grounds for presupposing that the beliefs are unchanging. You can have plenty of conflict of the most murderous kind without any accusations of witchcraft. The intensification of the practice of witchcraft in African cities during recent decades has produced no court proceedings against witches because officials regarded it all as a superstition. So we can infer nothing about the practice from the court records. All we know is that the fear spread, and people became more eager to search for witches and to punish them.

We must bear in mind that the changes in the European societies of the seventeenth century were very much slower than the upheaval wrought in the lives of African tribesmen by the impact of a fully-fledged industrial civilisation. And for this reason they could not have brought disorientation and uprooting on the same scale. We have, therefore, no grounds for even suspecting that the same causal link was involved. Some historians' love for the word 'Revolution' should not lead us to forget that economic changes in the previous centuries to which this label is often affixed (including the so-called Industrial Revolution) were so slow that they escaped the notice of most people who lived through them. We must conclude, therefore, that, though interesting and ingenious, Macfarlane's thesis offers no adequate explanation.

More plausible is H. R. Trevor-Roper's view[16] linking the Witch Craze with the Wars of Religion. Whereas the changes in the economy (other than natural calamities) were almost imperceptible, wars did bring violent shocks and upheavals, and evoked waves of emotion of an altogether different dimension from what might be generated by the slow processes of commercialisation of personal relations and disintegration of village solidarity. One can well imagine how, faced with devastation and slaughter, gripped by fear and inclined to look for scapegoats, superstitious people would succumb to an obsession with witches. And it is true that the biggest hunts occurred in Germany, which was more devastated by the wars than any other country.

On the other hand, the correspondence is only very broad – by country (in the sense of a cultural area) and epoch – and is not evident region-by-region and year-by-year, as many of the big Witch Hunts took place in regions unscourged by wars. Further-more, we cannot explain something unprecedented by something of much more common occurrence – many wars, just as sanguinary as those of the sixteenth and the seventeenth centuries, have been waged before, and since, without provoking Witch Hunts. Another weakness of this explanation is that no one has shown what the psychological mechanism would be which would link fighting and war with an obsession with witches. The soldiers of those times were habitual looters and rapists, inclined to maltreat all defenceless people. But why should they have wanted to burn women rather than merely abuse them? Nor do we have any grounds for supposing that the civilians must have become obsessed with fear of witches because they lived in fear of the soldiers. In most wars civilians were afraid of soldiers' depredations, but even at the height of the Witch Craze there is no evidence that anyone blamed witches for causing wars or the havoc wrought by these, although they were held responsible for disease. This is perfectly understand-able: people could see the soldiers killing, burning and looting – there was no mystery about it – but they knew nothing about bacteria.

Trevor-Roper's thesis could be defended by pointing out that he speaks of the Wars of Religion rather than wars pure and simple. But what are 'wars of religion'? The explanation clearly falls short if we mean thereby wars between collectivities holding different religions, because no one claims that the wars between the Christians and the Moslems or the Catholics and the Greek-

Orthodox provoked waves of witch hunting. However, the distinguishing feature which the historians have in mind when they
use the expression in question is wars accompanied by forcible
conversions or by extermination of heretics. Thus restricted, the
thesis becomes more defensible but remains, none the less, defective because there seems to be no co-variation before the sixteenth
century. One of the most ferocious wars of religion was the crusade
against the Albigenses in the thirteenth century; yet there is no
evidence that it was accompanied by witch hunts as distinct from
the persecution of the heretics. The same can be said about the
wars against the Hussites and the sanguinary suppression of the
Lollards by Henry V in the fifteenth century. At the other end (as
Kurt Baschwitz emphasises), witch trials went on after the Peace
of Westphalia.[17]

Like Stalin's chief prosecutor, Andrei Vishinsky, the Medieval
and Renaissance theologians and lawyers were unsparing in
heaping up reasons for a condemnation: witches were held to be
guilty of heresy in the shape of the pact with Satan, while heretics
were commonly accused of witchcraft and sexual vice, especially
sodomy and incest, as well as of theft, robbery, arson, poisoning
the wells and whatnot. The practice of burning people alive was
used extensively in Spain to force the conversion of Jews and
Moslems before it was employed in Witch Hunts. Spain, however,
never experienced the massive witch hunts of the kind that afflicted
northern Europe. Consequently, despite its prominent role in
many witch trials, we cannot regard the Inquisition as the sole
instigator in view of the fact that it rejected this role in the country
where it developed fastest and furthest. In any case, many more
persons were put to death for heresy than for witchcraft. To punish
someone for heresy there was no need to trump up charges on
another score. Why, then, should a suppression of heresy lead to
a hunt for witches?

Though indiscriminate in heaping up abuse, the persecutors
discriminated between witches and heretics in penal procedure.
Heretics could often save their skins by recantation and repentance
(as did Galileo) whereas to a witch this escape route was normally
closed. Heretics and rebels were very often burnt or impaled
summarily on flimsy evidence, without waiting for their confessions. This could be done because many of them had in fact done
or said what they were accused of. Extracting confessions through
torture was essential if witches were to be found at all, as there

could have been no proper evidence because the victims could not have done what they were accused of.

The weightiest argument against explaining Witch Hunts in terms of any form of 'struggle for power' stems from the predominance of women among the victims and the inclusion of a good number of children, which is exactly the contrary to what happens in wars and political or religious persecutions. Usually only men are killed, while women and children are enslaved or otherwise ill-used. With extremely few exceptions, not only the top leaders but also the lower-rank organisers and preachers of all religious or political movements noted in history have been men; which explains the aforementioned fact that repression has always been directed mainly at men. The Witch Hunters, in contrast, more often picked on women who, moreover, were commonly single and poor, or at least neither rich nor powerful, and therefore of all kinds of people were the least likely to represent a danger to the authorities. Soldan, Heppe and Bauer[18] give lists of victims of trials in various German cities. Among these about every fifteenth person is a child; e.g. a blind beggar girl aged eleven, two brothers aged ten and eleven, a shoemaker's apprentice aged thirteen. On the other hand, in the same series of trials, we also find a gravedigger aged forty-two, a mother of three children aged twenty-four, a single woman aged thirty-two, a burgomaster's wife and a priest of unspecified age. The two youngest victims were aged six and eight. With victims of this kind, it is completely implausible to interpret the Witch Hunts as some kind of a purge or repression of enemies. (We must also bear in mind that any form of such an interpretation contradicts flatly the explanations offered by Keith Thomas and Alan Macfarlane.)

A slight variant along the lines of a political explanation is the view (the most widely held among the British historians) that the Witch Hunts were the outcome of the momentum of the machinery of repression which, once set up by the Church for purpose of hunting heretics, went on grinding lesser deviants perhaps because the inquisitors found themselves with nothing to do once heresy had been stamped out but wanted to keep themselves in business. This explanation rests upon an implicit assumption that no other potential victims were available, and this is rather far-fetched. Even if they ran out of known heretics, why couldn't the inquisitors pick on suspects, sinners, usurers, or some ethnic or occupational category? Moreover it would be easy to find victims whose possessions were a little more substantial than what most people accused of witchcraft had. Persecutions of Jews often brought substantial booty, but witch hunts were only occasionally profitable, and then mostly only to low-grade personnel like executioners to whom a few odd household goods made a difference. So an economic motive for keeping the repression going can be ruled out. On the other hand, the explanation in terms of the momentum of repression does not fit the crucial fact of the shift in the sex ratio among the victims after 1500. After that date heretics continued to be mostly men whereas witches were mostly women. There are many historical examples of the machinery of terror acquiring a momentum of its own and overshooting the purpose for which it was set up – they range from the carnage launched by the ancient Chinese emperor Wu to Stalin's purges and the rule of Idi Amin in Uganda. In all such cases, however, the overwhelming majority of the victims were men. The shift in the sex ratio is unique.

The Protestants' addiction to witch-hunting provides an equally decisive argument against any explanation invoking the inertia of the institutions, because the Reformation consisted above all of the destruction of the hierarchic edifice of the Church, including the Inquisition. Owing to the absence of centralised control the Witch Hunts in Protestant lands tended to be grass-roots affairs (which, incidentally, may account for the difference between the findings of Mandrou and those of Thomas and Macfarlane); but obsessive fear was just as much in evidence. Luther, Calvin and their followers discarded many of the deeply-rooted tenets of the old Church but fully upheld the notions about witches.

Why? This agreement not only could not stem from but was actually contrary to their idea of going back to the Bible rather than accepting the Pope's and Bishops' decrees. The teachings of the New Testament are wholly opposed to sanguinary barbarities, and it disregards this particular superstition. True, the Old Testament mentions witches but only casually and it bears no trace of an obsession with danger from them. The sentence in the Old Testament 'thou shalt not suffer a witch alive' was constantly invoked by the witch hunters but could have been disregarded, like so many other pronouncements of the Bible (such as the injunction to offer the other cheek or the condemnation of acquisitiveness in the parable about the camel and the eye of a needle), particularly as it occurs only once and without any emphasis. In the Protestant theology the Saints were purged and the Virgin Mary demoted but the witches retained their recently augmented importance, despite the fact that the doctrinal justification for the persecutions was provided by the Catholic theologians whom Luther and Calvin execrated. In Scotland the bloodiest hunts were carried out by the Calvinist zealots following in the footsteps of John Knox; so that there the greatest carnage occurred after the destruction of the old machinery of repression. An explanation in terms of 'momentum' can, then, be dismissed. The concordance of attitudes between embattled enemies can cease to be shrouded in mystery only if we can discover circumstances which affected them all regardless of their affiliations and their hate for one another.

In his erudite and massive Ph.D. thesis (1977), submitted to the University of Reading under a snappy title, 'The Politics of Danger', Dr Ronald Vanelli presents witchcraft accusations as a scapegoating mechanism which off-loads tensions generated by conflicts which threaten some people's self-image, status and power. Although this work offers a unique comparative survey of persecutions almost throughout the world, and contains many valuable sidelights, its first defect is that it includes under this category affairs which have nothing to do with witchcraft in any tolerably precise meaning of this word. When some people dubbed the activities of Senator McCarthy a 'witch hunt', they wanted to suggest that the Soviet agents whom he proposed to uncover were a figment of his imagination like the nocturnal rides on broomsticks. However, even if we believed that, in fact, there had been no such agents in the USA, we still would have no reason for ruling out this possibility. In reality, some agents have been caught and there are good grounds for assuming that there must have been others who were never discovered. McCarthy might have been misguided about where and how to ferret them out and he may have deliberately exaggerated and sowed confusion about this matter. Nonetheless, it is completely misleading to take the metaphorical and tendentious dubbing of his activities as equivalent of a fear evoked by pure delusions.

The second defect of Vanelli's work is that it attempts to explain something which is far from ubiquitous by a factor which is, as in every human society there are struggles for esteem and power.

Nor is there any evidence that 'threats to self-image' were more common where persecutions of witches were taking place than elsewhere. The focus on dangers to esteem and self-esteem stems, I think, from a culturally self-centred outlook of a denizen of an affluent and well-medicated society, able to forget about the dangers which inspired the most pervasive fear in earlier times, as they still do in the less fortunate parts of the globe: famine and disease.

The word 'disease' provides the clue: but, before following it, we must glance at one more interpretation. Writing before the present fad and fashion of always seeking economic or political explanations, Margaret Murray[19] depicted the Witch Hunts as a repressive action of the Christian Churches against the remnants of the pre-Christian religions. Persons burnt as witches were, according to Murray, the priests and, above all, priestesses of the old religion. Their rituals were misrepresented and dubbed as witchcraft. The reunions, labelled 'Witches' Sabbaths', did in fact take place, although not in the form described by the demonologists but rather as regular worship of the old pagan gods. The numerical predominance of women among the victims is explained by their greater attachment to the tradition and the central role of home worship in the pre-Christian religions which had more priestesses than priests.

However, it seems highly implausible that the Church would have waited so many centuries – in the former domains of the Roman Empire more than a thousand years – before launching an attack on the pagan priesthoods. An even greater weakness stems from the assumption that there was a good deal of truth in the confessions. True, Margaret Murray and her followers rely on records from English courts where the most dreadful tortures employed on the Continent were not used. Nevertheless, the accused were locked up in cold, dark and damp dungeons; they were starved, deprived of sleep and beaten. Friedrich Spee, one of the brave opponents (whose book inaugurated the waning of the hunts and who had been a confessor of the accused), wrote: 'We would all have confessed to being witches if we hade been tortured.'[20]

Furthermore, many victims admitted flying on broomsticks, causing storms, and performing other impossible deeds. Why then should we assume that there must be some truth in what they said about acts which we deem possible? Under torture, many Jews have confessed to 'poisoning the wells', killing little Christian boys, and squeezing their blood into Passover bread. Following Murray's method we would have to assume that, because such deeds were physically possible, there must have been some truth in the confessions, despite the obvious untruth of the confessions about making Christ's blood flow by piercing the Eucharist with a knife or causing pestilence.

Keith Thomas, Jean Delumeau, and some other historians who have examined the same materials say that Margaret Murray and her followers make a very arbitrary selection of very late documents. As I have not studied these sources, I have no opinion on this matter; but it seems to me impossible that an organised religion could be widely practised for a thousand years without being detected and attacked by the Church until the sixteenth century. As a matter of fact, the pre-Christian religions were suppressed by Draconian punishments much earlier. Charlemagne slaughtered the pagan priests in Saxony. In the eleventh century there was a large uprising in Poland led by pagan priests which was drowned in blood. It might have been prompted by the dreadful punishments ordered by King Boleslaw the Valiant (Chrobry) for non-compliance with the rules of Christianity: such as pulling out teeth for eating meat on Fridays, or cutting off the tongue for blasphemy. There are records of campaigns against pagan priests in Scandinavia; but, they all took place soon after the implantation of Christianity. As there is no shred of evidence of a pagan threat to Christianity in the sixteenth century, Margaret Murray's thesis is untenable, particularly as the authors of demonological treatises speak of the plague of witches as something new.

When the old religions still posed a real threat the Church suppressed them ruthlessly, but without succumbing to a frenzy, relying on punishments which were harsh but not wildly sadistic:

In the seventh century was composed the *Liber Pœnitentialia* of S. Theodore, seventh Archbishop of Canterbury, the earliest collection of ecclesiastical disciplinary laws for England. No less than the whole of one section is concerned with magic practices and ceremonies, a penance being duly assigned for each offence. The thirty-seventh Book has as its rubric, 'Of Idolatry and Sacrilege, and of those who pay divine honours to certain Angels, and evil-doers, soothsayers, poisoners, charmers, diviners, and those who vow their vows otherwise than to Holy Church, and the man who on the Kalends of January goeth about in the masque of a stag or a bull calf, as also of astrologers, and those who by their craft raise storms.' There are six-and-twenty heads, and of these many are so important that the more significant provisions of the principal enactments must at least be given. 'If anyone sacrifices to demons, one year of penance if he be a clown of low estate, if he be of higher degree, 10 years. If anyone sacrifice a second or a third time to demons he shall do penance for 3 years. If anyone commits sacrilege, that is if he consulteth soothsayers who divine by birds or in any other forbidden way he shall do penance 3 years, and of these one shall he fast on bread and water. It is unlawful for any, cleric or layman, to exercise the craft of a seer or a charmer, or to make philtres, and all such as practice such arts or use them we order to be expelled from the church. If anyone by evil spells hath slain another . . . If anyone hath poisoned another from jealousy and yet hath not slain him . . . If anyone hath procured abortion . . . If anyone frequents seers, whom men call diviners, or hath practised any charms, for this is devilish . . . If anyone hath made a trial of those lots, which are wrongly called the Holy Lots, or hath cast any lots at all, or hath with evil intent cast lots, or hath divined . . . If any woman hath divined or hath used devilish evocations . . . If any woman hath placed her son or daughter upon the house-top or in the oven in order to ensure them health . . . If anyone hath burned wheat upon the spot where a man hath died in order to ensure the health and prosperity of his household . . . If anyone in order to ensure health to his young son hath passed the baby upwards through some cavity in the earth, and then hath closed fast the hole behind him with thorns and brambles . . . anyone who hath had resource to diviners and cleaveth to the traditions of the heathen, or hath brought men of this craft into his house in order to find out some secret by their evil science, or in order to expiate some wrong . . . If anyone hath vowed a vow and hath fulfilled the same at a clump of trees, or a spring of water, or at certain rocks, or at a spot where boundaries meet, or at any other place whatsoever, save in God's house, the church, he shall do penance fasting on bread and water for 3 years, since this is sacrilege, and verily devilish. Who hath eaten or drunk in honour of idols one year shall he do penance fasting on bread and water. If anyone at the Kalends of January goeth about as a stag or a bull-calf, that is, making himself into a wild animal, and dressing in the skins of a herd animal, and putting on the heads of beasts; those who in such wise transform themselves into the appearance of a wild animal, let them to penance for three years, because this is devilish.'[21]

In view of the fact that all the hitherto advanced explanations are either inadequate or simply false, as well as mutually contradictory, we would be faced with a complete mystery if no more plausible explanation could be devised. I contend, however, that there is an explanation which fits the data much better than any of the preceding and subsumes those of their points which retain some validity.

THE FATAL CLUE

The inclination to seek the causes of illness in witchcraft is by no means a peculiarity of Europeans in early modern times but an almost universal (if not absolutely universal) feature of all pre-scientific cultures, although the role of witchcraft varies greatly in details and importance. While the Pygmies of the Congo pay scant attention to witchcraft, the Azande (to take another African example) see in it the cause of all illness. The Europeans of the sixteenth century did not go so far as the Azande and, acquainted with the works of Hippocrates through the writings of Galen, they conceived of other causes of disease such as bad air or food. However, even the most enlightened of them (who regarded the stories of witches flying on broomsticks and feasting with Satan as fairy tales) did not deny that illness *could* be caused by witchcraft. To understand their outlook we must bear in mind that, as scientific medicine did not yet exist, there were no compelling reasons for excluding this possibility. Indeed, the practice of medicine was still thoroughly mixed up with magic. Given the state of knowledge and the nature of the beliefs, it was inevitable that any epidemic would fan the fear of witches and prompt a multiplication of suspicions, accusations and persecutions. The epidemic which coincided chronologically with the Witch Craze was that of syphilis.

Syphilis was either brought to Europe by the sailors of Columbus or underwent a mutation at the beginning of the sixteenth century which greatly increased its virulence. Perhaps a milder strain existed in the Old World before a more powerful variant was brought from America. Be this as it may, there is no doubt that there was a terrible epidemic from the beginning of the sixteenth century until the second half of the seventeenth century. Innumerable sources bear ample witness to the havoc it wrought and the dread it inspired. It was known from the beginning that it was transmitted through copulation. The following extract from an entry on The Harlot in an anonymous book called *The Profane State*, published during the reign of Charles I, illustrates the common notions:

> *She* [the harlot] *dieth commonly of a lothsome disease.* I mean that disease, unknown to Antiquity, created within some hundreds of years, which took the name from Naples. When hell invented new degrees in sinnes, it was time for heaven to invent new punishments. Yet is this new disease now grown so common and ordinary, as if they meant to put divine Justice to a second task to find out a newer. And now it is high time for our Harlot, being grown lothsome to her self, to runne out of her self by repentance.
>
> Some conceive that when King Henrie the eighth destroyed the publick Stews in this Land (which till his time stood on the banks side on Southwark next the Bear-garden, beasts and beastly women being very fit neighbours) he rather scattered than quenched the fire of lust in this kingdome, and by turning the flame out of the chimney where it had a vent, more endangered the burning of the Commonwealth. But they are deceived: for whilst the Laws of the Land tolerated open uncleannesse, God might justly have made the whole State do penance for whoredome; whereas now that sinne though committed, yet not permitted, and though (God knows) it be too generall, it is still but personall.

Although it might have been counter productive rather than helpful for avoiding contagion, and must have had deleterious effects on health in other ways, the closing of public baths is a measure of the fear of syphilis. Medieval towns had public baths where all orders of society (or almost all) were wont to go and wallow collectively, male and female naked together. These became very rare or disappeared altogether. For example, in Frankfurt, which had forty such establishments in 1400, there were only nine in 1530. In the same period, wooden bathtubs disappeared from inns and hotels throughout Europe. Only in Finland and in Budapest under the Ottoman rule did the public town-baths survive. The public baths which came into existence in France in the late seventeenth century (that is, when the epidemic of syphilis was on the wane) were public only in the sense that anyone could go in for a high fee – which meant that they were available only to the rich – but the bathing was individual.[22]

An illness caught through sin, which was not only fatal but also repulsive, would inevitably evoke harrowing feelings of shame, guilt, and rage against the partner presumed to have transmitted the disease. The psychological mechanism of generalisation and stereotyping would tend to produce in the sufferers a hostile attitude to the other sex, which through imitation and the stimulus of generalised fear would spread among healthy individuals as well. Furthermore, according to psychoanalytic theory, the stronger the feelings of guilt, the more likely they are to be projected – that is repressed from consciousness and imputed to others. The belief in witchcraft constituted a particularly suitable vehicle for such a projection, permitting a displacement of the feelings of guilt by a grievance about being bewitched. These mechanisms would operate in women as well as men; but men ruled and therefore their inclinations determined the course of events.

Crucially important was the fact that public opinion was moulded chiefly by the clergy, who were under the obligation to lead exemplary lives and in the Catholic Church to observe chastity. They therefore had reason to feel guilt and shame with special poignancy and would be particularly prone to seek scapegoats on whom these feelings could be projected, and who could be sacrificed in expiation. The strength of these feelings would fuel the mental mechanism of generalisation and stereotyping through which the hate against the partner, from whom the disease might have been contracted, would be extended to others. In principle, the process of generalisation of attitudes can operate upon any common feature. But, here, since all the resentment came from the consequences of the sexual act, the stereotype would be naturally extended to the entire opposite sex, while the most defenceless members thereof would be most likely to be picked on as scapegoats.

To repeat, there is no reason to suppose that this mechanism did not operate among women. It is very likely that the epidemic of syphilis did evoke among women a groundswell of resentment against men, particularly perhaps against the priests and monks who abused their influence to lead them into sin. Perhaps if the women had had more power, there would have been more male victims of Witch Hunts, but since all the power lay in men's hands, only they were able to give vent to their desire to find scapegoats. It is possible, nevertheless, that some trials of men – especially of clergymen – were instigated by women. The famous affair of Loudun in France in the middle of the seventeenth century appears to be an example. As I said earlier, there are ample grounds for rejecting the view that Witch Trials were a consciously employed method of subjugating women. Nevertheless, the extent to which one sex can inflict sufferings on the other must reflect their relative power, even when the motives and actions are irrational and self-damaging. We might, therefore, take the sex ratio of the victims as a rough indication of the imbalance of power between the sexes. It was the sexual nature of the disease that directed the search for scapegoats against women, while during other plagues religious or ethnic minorities suffered. (The outbreaks of bubonic plague were regularly followed by massacres of Jews.)

The more defenceless an individual the more likely he or she is to be picked on as a scapegoat. Thus, in the patrilineal and patriarchal tribes of Africa more accusations are levelled against women than against men – which is not the case in the matrilineal tribes. This does not mean that such accusations are a deliberate method of 'keeping women down', which would presuppose that the men do not truly believe in witchcraft. In many tribes in Africa and elsewhere, deliberate tricks are employed for keeping the women under control by so-called secret societies – secret not in the sense that their existence or membership is secret but only that they keep secrets. One of these is that they imitate the voice of the spirit with a device known as a bull-roarer. When this spirit wanders about the village all women and girls as well as uninitiated boys must hide, and any of them who peeps out is killed on the spot. Any initiated man who divulged this secret to a woman or an uninitiated boy would also be killed. Since the initiated men can see one of their number twirling the bull-roarer, they must be aware that they are perpetrating a deliberate trick, although even here they can delude themselves that the spirit enters the bull-roarer. As far as witchcraft is concerned, all evidence suggests that the belief in its efficacity and the fear were as a rule genuine.

The ground for attacks against women when syphilis struck was prepared by the change in the attitude towards them which took place during the two preceding centuries, and which Jean Delumeau calls 'demonisation.' Although there is no trace of it in the sayings of Jesus Christ, the idea that women are a source of evil has been present in the Christian tradition at least since St Augustine, and formed a part of the cluster of values which extolled chastity and deprecated pleasures of the flesh. This attitude, however, underwent a drastic reinforcement during the fourteenth and fifteenth centuries and reached a frenzy during the sixteenth. The latter change lends force to my thesis but the reinforcement during the fourteenth and fifteenth centuries calls for another explanation – which can be found if we look at the tightening-up on celibacy of the clergy and the multiplication of the monastic orders which occurred during that time. The connection between the two trends is perfectly understandable in the light of psychiatry. The more stringent observance of chastity would cause the priests and monks to be more tormented by carnal desire. The aggressive impulses generated by this frustration would be directed at the objects of desire, while the repressed feelings of guilt (for indulging in sinful thoughts or acts) would (through a process of projection) lead to imputation of evil proclivities to all women, above all of wanting to tempt, tease and lead holy men to perdition.[23]

The advance of sacerdotal celibacy stretched over a thousand years: from the Synod of 384 which advised the higher ranks of the clergy to remain celibate (without, however, prescribing any punishment for non-compliance) to the Counter-Reformation when celibacy began to be enforced effectively. Important steps were taken by the Synods during the eleventh and twelfth centuries which prohibited the sons of priests taking over their fathers' offices, and later excluded them altogether from entering the priesthood. Married priests were forbidden to celebrate mass. In 1139 the Lateran Council declared marriages of the higher clergy invalid, and penalised married priests of the lower orders by depriving them of benefices and legal immunities.[24] After the fourth Lateran Council in 1215, through the tireless vigilance of Innocent III, open marriage of priests ceased except in outlying regions where inspection was difficult. This, however, did not mean that chastity was observed. This is what the nineteenth century historian Henry C. Lea says on the subject of concubinage:

> However deplorable such an alternative might be in itself, it was
> surely preferable to the mischief which the unquenched and
> ungoverned passions of a pastor might inflict upon his parish;
> and the instances of this were too numerous and too glaring to
> admit of much hesitation in electing between the two evils.
> Even Gerson, the leader of mystic ascetics, who recorded his
> unbounded admiration for the purity of celibacy in his *Dialogus
> Naturae et Sophiae de Castitate Clericorum*, saw and appreciated its
> practical evils, and had no scruple in recommending concubinage
> as a preventive, which, though scandalous in itself, might serve
> to prevent greater scandals. It therefore requires no great stretch
> of credulity to believe the assertion of Sleidan, that in some of
> the Swiss Cantons it was the custom to oblige a new pastor, on
> entering upon his functions, to select a concubine, as a necessary
> protection to the virtue of his female parishioners, and to the
> peace of the families entrusted to his spiritual direction. Indeed,
> we have already seen (p. 261), on the authority of Council of
> Valladolid in 1322, that such a practice was not uncommon in
> Spain.

Lea goes on to emphasise:

> In thus reviewing the influences which a nominally celibate
> clergy exercised over those entrusted to their care, it is perhaps
> scarcely too much to conclude that they were largely responsible
> for the laxity of morals which is a characteristic of mediaeval
> society. No one who has attentively examined the records left
> to us of that society can call in question the extreme prevalence
> of the licentiousness which everywhere infected it. Christianity
> had arisen as the great reformer of a world utterly corrupt. How
> earnestly its reform was directed to correcting sexual immorality
> is visible in the persistence with which the Apostles condemned
> and forbade a sin that the Gentiles scarcely regarded as a sin. The
> early Church was consequently pure, and its very asceticism is
> a measure of the energy of its protest against the all-pervading
> licence which surrounded it. Its teachings, as we have seen,
> remained unchanged. Fornication continued to be a mortal sin,
> yet the period of its unquestioned domination over the conscience
> of Europe was the very period in which licence among the

Teutonic races was most unchecked. A Church which, though founded on the Gospel, and wielding the illimitable power of the Roman hierarchy, could yet allow the feudal principle to extend to the *'jus primae noctis'* or *'droit de marquette'* and whose ministers in their character of temporal seigneurs could even occasionally claim the disgusting right themselves, was evidently exercising its influence not for good but for evil.[25]

(Lea is referring here to the right of the Lord to have the bride of his serf for the first night.) It was not until the sixteenth century and, finally, at the Council of Trent (1545–1563) that the final curbs were put on concubinage; thenceforth unchastity of priests and monks had to be clandestine, and it appears to have become much rarer. It is usually said that the new strictness was a response to the Protestant challenge. This is on the whole true; but the impact of syphilis must have played an important part in this change. In the preceding chapter I have given reasons for linking the rise of puritanism as well as the introduction of a stronger dose of Puritanism, in the wider sense, into the Catholic Church, with the epidemic. Here I should like to add that it must have made the obligation of chastity much easier to enforce because sinners would be likely to be detected by the visible symptoms of the disease.

It appears, therefore, that the lay clergy began to suffer from serious sexual frustration only in the sixteenth century. None the less, chastity was becoming more widely practised in earlier times because the three preceding centuries saw the great multiplication of the monastic orders and the tightening up of the discipline on this score within them. Indeed, the monks were the chief helpers of the Popes in their struggle to impose celibacy on the lay clergy. And as for the 'demonisation' of women, we must remember that before 1500 nearly all writers and all theologians were monks.

An objection to the foregoing argument might be raised on the ground that although their clergy were allowed to marry, the Protestants also burned witches. The thesis, however, can be saved by taking into account the following considerations.

The first is that the Catholics burned more witches than the Protestants: at least twice or three times as many. Secondly, the demonisation of women had gone very far by the time of the Reformation; and the Protestants inherited this tradition. Thirdly, the Protestant theologians shared with the Catholics the anti-hedonist principles. They abolished celibacy of the clergy not because they approved of indulgence in pleasures but as a way of stopping fornication. The abolition of confessions and absolutions, moreover, made it more difficult to get rid of feelings of guilt. We can plausibly surmise that this factor would tend to foster 'projection' and 'scapegoating', and would counteract in some measure the contrary effects of the abolition of celibacy. A much stricter enforcement of premarital chastity and marital fidelity – in combination with the puritanical refusal ever to discuss matters pertaining to sexual intercourse – would also tend to generate enough hang-ups to stimulate demonisation of women. Furthermore, the absence of a powerful hierarchy made the Protestant clergy more vulnerable to castigation by their own flock for not living up to what they preached. Thus, any sign of having caught syphilis might bring upon a Protestant clergyman an even prompter punishment than in the case of a Catholic. None the less, although John Calvin and other Protestant theologians supported the hunts for witches, the chief theorists of the persecution were all Catholics and nearly all were monks. Monks played a crucial role in nearly all the hunts which took place in the Catholic lands, the Dominicans being particularly prominent.

The Witch Craze did not spread to the lands of the Orthodox Church: neither Russia nor the principalities of Wallachia and Moldavia were affected. The ferocious persecution of the Old Believers in Russia was accompanied by no witch hunts – which provides another argument against the view that they were a by-product of a fight against heresies. The schism between the Eastern and Western Churches occurred before the celibacy of the clergy was established; and the Orthodox priests continued to marry. As the schism occurred several centuries before the demonisation of women reached a high pitch in the West, the Eastern Church was not affected by this tradition, in contrast to the Protestant denominations. True, the Orthodox bishops were celibate, but they normally underwent voluntary castration before promotion; an entrant into the priesthood had a choice between ambition and marriage. Being castrated, the higher clergy of the Orthodox Church could not have suffered so much from frustration and guilt as did their Western equivalents. Consequently, there must have been less scope within their minds for the operations of the mechanisms of projection and scapegoating, which underlay the demonisation of women and the Witch Hunt in the West.

The same factor explains why the Witch Craze never spread to the lands of Islam, where the mullahs were hardly likely to suffer from severe sexual frustration as they usually had many wives. Furthermore, you cannot demonise women when their position is so low that they are little more than chattels. Cloistered in purdah, covered up by chadors and yashmaks from head to foot, women could hardly be seen as temptresses by polygamous Moslem theologians.

Nor did the Witch Craze infect the Jews, although they were close witnesses of these happenings. Significantly, from the viewpoint of the present thesis, rabbis are not only allowed but are obliged to marry: even a widowed rabbi will not be accepted by his community unless he remarries.

It is likely that the proportion of priests and monks who were suffering from severe sexual frustration was much greater when entry into their ranks was the only avenue to freedom from want and a respectable status for men of humble origin. Many younger sons of better-off families were forced to take the vows against their will, and only in an ecclesiastic career could a man of intellectual disposition find an opportunity to devote himself to study. When it became possible to attain either of these goals in other walks of life, the entrants would be more self-selected in respect of their tolerance of chastity, that is, a weaker sexual appetite. Psychoanalytic theory suggests that lesser sexual frustration would diminish the inclination to demonise women.[26]

By taking into account the factors of celibacy and puritanism we can explain the rarity and lesser ferocity of the persecutions in England, where the writings on the subject also lacked the florid extravagance of the continental treatises. The abolition of sacerdotal celibacy was one of the first steps in Henry VIII's breach with Rome but (in contrast to the schism between the Greek and the Roman Churches) this event occurred well after the implantation of the fear of women. Consequently, the Church of England was not immune to the craze. However, its lesser proclivity in this direction can be explained by the fact that it was less puritanical than other Protestant denominations, especially the Church of Scotland where the persecution was just as intense as in Germany. England was also affected by the general current of puritanism (prompted, as we saw earlier, by the epidemic of syphilis) but this current was somewhat dampened by the character of the Reformation in England where it was imposed from above by a licentious king, and was never a mass movement led by a crowd-

swayer like Luther or Knox who could only resist the power of
Rome by inspiring mass fervour. The Anglican clergy, moreover,
were tied to the aristocracy and the gentry who were much less
predisposed to abstemiousness than the hard-working classes, and
therefore less susceptible to Puritan preaching. The combined effect
of the abolition of celibacy and the lesser involvement with
puritanism, made the Anglican clergy less exposed to the torments
of guilt feelings and therefore less inclined to demonise women
than their Catholic, Calvinist or even Lutheran counterparts. It
was not until the nineteenth century that the English and their
clergy became more puritanical and prudish than other Protestant
nations, but by then other factors ruled out a witch craze, and the
sexual hang-ups could manifest themselves only in minor forms
of misogynism like the exclusion of women from clubs and pubs,
and a greater amount of segregation of the sexes at dinner parties
than was customary in other countries of northern Europe.

In view of the foregoing considerations it is not surprising that
more people were put to death as witches in England during the
short period of the Puritan rule than during the long domination
of the Anglican Church.

Although they were unable to explain them, many historians
have commented on the aforementioned peculiarities of English
history. The great Victorian historian Lecky did offer an explanation
by attributing them to the English heritage of political freedom and
individualism, but this interpretation cannot be reconciled with
the surge of persecutions during the rule by the Puritans, whose
ecclesiastic institutions were much more individualistic and democratic than the Church of England. Lecky noted these facts but
drew no inference. Furthermore, local autonomy, individualism
(whether economic or religious) and freedoms of various kinds
developed much further in the American colonies than in England,
where the persecution of witches ceased sooner. Indeed the trials
in Salem, New England, became famous precisely because they
took place when in England such events already belonged to the
past. An explanation of this time lag is not far to seek: New
England was ruled by the Puritans.

OF LUST AND DISEASE

The sources bear ample witness to the preoccupation of the Witch Hunters with lust and disease. The Emperor Maximilian I, who, in 1495, declared syphilis to be God's punishment for men's sins, became very worried about depredations caused by witches. In 1508 he sought advice on this matter from Abbot Trithemius, who in that year published a book called *The Enemy of Witchcraft*. There he wrote:

> It is a repulsive breed, that of the witches, especially the female among them, who, with the help of evil spirits or magic potions, bring to mankind endless harm . . . Mostly they make people possessed by demons and let them be tormented by unheard of pains . . . Hearken, they even indulge in carnal intercourse with demons . . . Unfortunately, the number of these witches is very great, and even in the smallest village you can find a witch . . . People and cattle die through the wickedness of these women and nobody understands that it all comes from witches. Many people suffer most dreadful illnesses and do not know that they are bewitched.[27]

This passage, incidentally, suggests that the theologians were even more inclined than the common folk to attribute disease to witchcraft. Writing seventy years later, Jean Bodin declares:

> there are fifty women witches to one man. This happens, in my opinion, not in consequence of the weakness of this sex, because we can see untamable stubbornness in most of them . . . It would be more correct to say that it is the force of bestial lust which pushes the woman to these extremes in order to assuage her desires or to take revenge.[28]

Equally eloquent in linking lust and disease with witchcraft is the most influential manual of witch hunters, *The Hammer of Witches* (*Malleus Maleficarum*) written by two German monks, Jacobus Sprenger and Heinrich Krämer, alias Insistoris.[29] Here are a few quotations:

> All witchcraft comes from carnal lust, which is in women insatiable, these women satisfy their filthy lusts not only in

themselves, but even in the mighty ones of the age, of whatever state and condition; causing by all sorts of witchcraft the death of their souls through the excessive infatuation of carnal love, in such a way that for no shame or persuasion can they desist from such acts.

. . . these wretches furthermore afflict and torment men and women, beasts of burthen, herd-beasts, as well as animals of other kinds, with terrible and piteous pains and sore diseases, both internal and external; they hinder men from performing the sexual act and women from conceiving, whence husbands cannot know their wives nor wives receive their husbands.

. . . when girls have been corrupted, and have been scorned by their lovers after they have immodestly copulated with them in the hope and promise of marriage with them and have found themselves disappointed in all their hopes and everywhere despised, they turn to the help and protection of devils; either for the sake of vengeance by bewitching those lovers or the wives they have married, or for the sake of giving themselves up to every sort of lechery. Alas! experience tells us that there is no number to such girls, and consequently the witches that spring from this class are innumerable.

Although far more women are witches than men, as was shown in the First Part of the work, yet men are more often bewitched than women. And the reason for this lies in the fact that God allows the devil more power over the venereal act, by which the original sin is handed down, than over the other human actions.

General acceptance of the notion that men are bewitched more often than women might have been helped by the fact that men succumb to syphilitic psychoses more often than women. As might be expected, Sprenger and Krämer took a dim view of the nature of love:

Philocaption, or inordinate love of one person for another, can be caused in three ways. Sometimes it is due merely to lack of control over the eyes; sometimes to the temptation of devils; sometimes to the spells of necromancers and witches, with the help of devils.

Not unlike other demonologists, our authors displayed great flights of imagination on the subjects of sexual relations between witches and devils.

> . . . our principal subject is the carnal act which Incubi in an assumed body perform with witches: unless perhaps anyone doubts whether modern witches practise such abominable coitus; and whether witches had their origin in this abomination.

> For it was possible for the devils to lie down themselves by the side of the sleeping husbands, during the time when a watch was being kept on the wives, just as if they were sleeping with their husbands.

> . . . to return to the question whether witches had their origin in these abominations, we shall say that they originated from some pestilent mutual association with devils, as is clear from our first knowledge of them. But no one can affirm with certainty that they did not increase and multiply by means of these foul practices, although devils commit this deed for the sake not of pleasure but of corruption. And this appears to be the order of the process. A Succubus devil draws the semen from a wicked man; and if he is that man's own particular devil, and does not wish to make himself an Incubus to a witch, he passes that semen on to the devil deputed to a woman or witch; and this last, under some constellation that favours his purpose that the man or woman so born should be strong in the practice of witchcraft, becomes the Incubus to the witch.

The following passage illustrates how a superstition could be reinforced by delusion or deceit.

> Husbands have actually seen Incubus devils swiving with their wives, although they have thought that they were not devils but men. And when they had taken up a weapon and tried to run them through, the devil has suddenly disappeared, making himself invisible. And then their wives have thrown their arms about them, although they have sometimes been hurt, and railed at their husbands, mocking them and asking them if they had eyes, or whether they were possessed of devils.

. . . these Incubus devils will not only infest those women who have been generated by means of such abominations, or those who have been offered to them by mid-wives, but that they try with all their might, by means of witches who are bawds or hot whores, to seduce all the devout and chaste maidens in that whole district or town.

With the exception, therefore, of these three classes of [holy] men, no one is secure from witches. For all others are liable to be bewitched, or to be tempted and incited by some witchery.

. . . in times long past the Incubus devils used to infest women against their wills. But the theory that modern witches are tainted with this sort of diabolic filthiness is not substantiated only in our opinion, since the expert testimony of the witches themselves, has made all these things credible; and that they do not now, as in times past, subject themselves unwillingly, but willingly embrace this most foul and miserable servitude.

The authors blame the evils of the world on women, remarking plaintively:

. . . for this age is dominated by women . . . and when the world is now full of adultery, especially among the most highly born; when all this is considered, I say, of what use is it to speak of remedies to those who desire no remedy?

As for the following passages, they lend particularly strong support to my thesis because all the effects of witchcraft listed by the authors fall under the headings of disturbances of the reproductive functions, other related illnesses and insanity!

. . . apart from the methods by which they injure other creatures, they have six ways of injuring humanity. And one is, to induce an evil love in a man for a woman, or in a woman for a man. The second is to plant hatred or jealousy in anyone. The third is to bewitch them so that a man cannot perform the genital act with a woman, or conversely a woman with a man; or by various means to procure an abortion, as has been said before. The fourth is to cause some disease in any of the human organs. The fifth, to take away life. The sixth, to deprive them of reason.

How witches impede and prevent the power of procreation . . . when they directly prevent the erection of the member which is accommodated to fructification. And this need not seem impossible, when it is considered that they are able to vitiate the natural use of any member. Secondly, when they prevent the flow of the vital essences to the members in which resides the motive force, closing up the seminal ducts so that it does not reach the generative vessels, or so that it cannot be ejaculated, or is fruitlessly spilled.

How, as it were, they deprive man of his virile member . . . A similar experience is narrated by a certain venerable Father from the Dominican House of Spires, well known in the Order for the honesty of his life and for his learning. 'One day,' he says, 'while I was hearing confessions, a young man came to me and, in the course of his confession, woefully said that he had lost his member. Being astonished at this, and not being willing to give it easy credence, since in the opinion of the wise it is a mark of light-heartedness to believe too easily, I obtained proof of it when I saw nothing on the young man's removing his clothes and showing the place. Then, using the wisest counsel I could, I asked whether he suspected anyone of having so bewitched him. And the young man said that he did suspect someone, but that she was absent and living in Worms. Then I said: I advise you to go to her as soon as possible and try your utmost to soften her with gentle words and promises, and he did so. For he came back after a few days and thanked me, saying that he was whole and had recovered everything. And I believed his words, but again proved them by the evidence of my eyes.'

Nor was the evidence for a misogynist persecution mania unrecorded:

. . . witches who in this way sometimes collect male organs in great numbers, as many as twenty or thirty members together, and put them in a bird's nest, or shut them up in a box, where they move themselves like living members.

In Ratisbon, a man was being tempted by the devil in the form of a woman to copulate, and became greatly disturbed when the devil would not desist. But it came into the poor man's mind that he ought to defend himself by taking Blessed Salt, as he had heard in a sermon. So he took some Blessed Salt on entering the bath-room; and the woman looked fiercely at him and cursing whatever devil had taught him to do this, suddenly disappeared. For the devil can, with God's permission, present himself either in the form of a witch, or by possessing the body of an actual witch . . . Some are protected against all sorts of witchcrafts, so that they can be hurt in no way; and others are particularly rendered chaste by the good Angels with regard to the generative function.

Similarly, St Gregory, in the first book of his *Dialogues*, tells of the Blessed Abbot Equitius. This man, he says, was in his youth greatly troubled by the provocation of the flesh; but the very distress of his temptation made him all the more zealous in his application to prayer. And when he continuously prayed Almighty God for a remedy against this affliction, an Angel appeared to him one night and seemed to make him a eunuch, and it seemed to him in his vision that all feeling was taken away from his genital organs; and from that time he was such a stranger to temptation as if he had no sex in his body.

My final quotation reveals the authors' hankering after a release from the torments of sexual frustration through castration (as was permitted in the Eastern Church):

Again, in the *Lives of the Fathers* collected by that very holy man St Heraclides, in the book which he calls *Paradise*, he tells of a certain holy Father, a monk named Helias. This man was moved by pity to collect thirty women in a monastery, and began to rule over them. But after two years, when he was thirty years old, he fled from the temptation of the flesh into a hermitage, and fasting there for two days, prayed to God, saying: 'O Lord God, either slay me, or deliver me from this temptation.' And in the evening a dream came to him, and he saw three Angels approach him; they asked him why he had fled from that Monastery of virgins. But when he did not dare to answer, for shame, the Angels said: If you are set free from temptation, will you return to your care of those women? And he answered that he would willingly. They then exacted an oath to that effect from him, and made him a eunuch. For one seemed to hold his hands, another his feet, and the third cut out his testicles with a knife; though this was not really so, but only seemed to be. And when they asked if he felt himself remedied, he answered that he was entirely delivered. So, on the fifth day he returned to the sorrowing women and ruled over them for the forty years that he continued to live, and never again felt a spark of that first temptation.

No less a benefit do we read to have been conferred upon the Blessed Thomas, a Doctor of our Order, whom his brothers imprisoned for entering that Order; and, wishing to tempt him, they sent him a seductive and sumptuously adorned harlot. But when the Doctor had looked at her, he ran to the material fire, and snatching up a lighted torch, drove the engine of the fire of lust out of his prison; and, prostrating himself in a prayer for the gift of chastity, went to sleep. Two Angels then appeared to him, saying: Behold, at the bidding of God we gird you with a girdle of chastity, which cannot be loosed by any other such temptation; neither can it be acquired by the merits of human virtue, but it is given as a gift by God alone. And he felt himself girded, and was aware of the touch of the girdle, and cried out and awaked. And thereafter he felt himself endowed with so great a gift of chastity, that from that time he abhorred all the delights of the flesh, so that he could not even speak to a woman except under compulsion, but was strong in his perfect chastity.

The date of publication of *Malleus* (1486), which was several years before the panic about syphilis spread, might be seen as an argument against linking Witch Hunting with the epidemic. I do not believe that this is so. At any particular time there are a number of eccentrics who attempt to propagate all kinds of out-of-the-way opinions. Although even what can be conceived by deviants is broadly limited by the culture in which they live, the narrower determination of beliefs by general circumstances occurs mainly on the level of selection through which some notions are given wide currency while others are consigned to insignificance or oblivion. The arrival of syphilis coincided with a radical change in the reception of *Malleus*. The first printing in 1486 was opposed by the clergy and was carried out with the help of a forged letter of approval. When Sprenger died in 1495 in Cologne he was buried without a mass. Krämer was expelled from more than one place by the local ecclesiastical authorities; he was suspended, and rehabilitated only in 1495 which happened to be the same year in which Emperor Maximilian bewailed the arrival of the new disease. Krämer was given a Papal commission in 1500 and died as an inquisitor in 1505. Their book was reissued sixteen times in Germany, eleven times in France, and twice in Italy. It had six editions in England between 1584 and 1669.

There is an analogy in respect of the time lag between the reception of *Malleus* and of *Mein Kampf* which Hitler published in 1924 but which attracted little attention until the panic and despair generated by the economic collapse of 1930.

In a book published in 1560 Pierre Boaistuau[30] records this attribution of physical deformities to sexual misdemeanours:

> It is certain that most often these monstrous creatures come from God's judgment, justice, punishment and curse, which permit that fathers and mothers produce such monstrosities through their horrible sins, as they rush indiscriminately like stupid beasts wherever their lust leads them without regard to time or place or other laws ordained by nature.

In a few cases I have come across – and I am confident that many more could be found by specialists who examined the sources from this angle – the reference to venereal disease is pretty obvious. Soldan, Heppe and Bauer, for example, report a trial of a prior's housekeeper who was accused by two priests of having caused through witchcraft their 'illness in the most secret parts of the body.'

In the plea for action he made in England, Bishop Jewel refers to sufferings which correspond to the symptoms of syphilis. According to Montague Summers:[31]

> His discourse against witches seems to have been delivered some time between November 1559 and 17 March 1560, probably in February of the latter year. At this time the ecclesiastical and civil authorities were in close touch, and no doubt the way was being laid for drastic legislation on the subject of sorcery. A sermon delivered by a famous court preacher, a newly made Bishop, would carry great weight. And Jewel vehemently urged immediate action. It was, he told the Queen, 'the horrible using of your poor subjects' that forced him to be round and plain.

'This kind of people (I mean witches and sorcerers) within these few last years are marvellously increased within this Your Grace's realm. These eyes have seen most evident and manifest marks of their wickedness. Your Grace's subjects pine away even unto death, their colour fadeth, their flesh rotteth, their speech is benumbed, their senses are bereft. Wherefore, Your poor subjects' most humble petition unto Your Highness is, that the laws touching such malefactors may be put in due execution.'

Strype certainly says that this sermon was the occasion of the law passed in the fifth year of Elizabeth's reign, by which Witchcraft was again made a felony, as it had been in the reign of Henry VIII.

It seems odd that modern historians prate about economic and political bases when the treatises of witch-finders hardly refer to such matters but are full of pronouncements about lust, copulation, and disease. The monastic theologians displayed vivid imagination on the subject of witches and devils' sexual activities or the torments which lascivious people will suffer in hell. One of the favourite themes was how sinful women are punished on the organs used for sinning. A good deal of attention was given to the large size of the devil's penis, the swiftness with which he can alternate between intromission and cunnilinctus, or the witches' manner of kissing him on the anus.

An explanation of a pattern of behaviour may refer to circumstances unknown to the doers, but it ought at the same time to account for what they keep on saying: in this case why the writers who provided the justification of witch-hunting went on and on about sexual intercourse and disease, and why they advocated remedies involving prurient sadism. All this becomes easy to understand in the light of a psychoanalytic interpretation of the consequences of celibacy and syphilis.

Syphilis must have also stimulated witchcraft accusations in another way. It made them useful as a quite rational method of disavowing sin, and disclaiming responsibility for the visible and shaming symptoms which could be attributed to being bewitched instead of having engaged in illicit copulation. Such an explanation of one's sufferings would not only make it easier to avoid being blamed, despised and punished, but would also alleviate painful feelings of guilt and shame. As the ecclesiastics were enjoined to live in celibacy, if they were Catholics, or in exemplary monogamy, if they were Protestants, they had most to gain by availing themselves of the possibility of explaining their illness as due to a cause other than sin, and therefore, they would be particularly inclined to make strenuous efforts to convince everybody, including themselves, of the reality of occult causes of disease. However, as the spread of puritanism aggravated the moral and material penalties for sins of the flesh, laymen too would be increasingly attracted to a belief with afforded them a respectable explanation of unavowable sufferings. As women would be more severely punished and despised for unchastity, and inclined to feel shame and guilt more poignantly than men, they would be even more attracted to the belief which undermined the major premises for an imputation of guilt. And we must bear in mind that not only the actual sufferers would be attracted to this belief but also their friends, relatives and well-wishers as well as all those in whose minds lurked the fear that one day they too might need this excuse. There would be a snowballing effect because the lies and self-deceptions of some would be taken as information by others, who would treat it as particularly reliable if it came from people held in reverence. And the more such notions spread, the easier it would be for people to convince others as well as themselves to this effect and reinforce the superstitions of others.

Unable to do anything effective but none the less obliged to offer their services to make a living, the physicians must have also been attracted to the magical explanation of illnesses which would camouflage their ignorance and impotence. This was the view of Johannes Weyer, the courageous Dutch physician who opposed the mania and managed to escape the stake. In his book against the hunts which was condemned by James I along with Reginald Scot's work, he wrote: 'ignorant and unskilful physicians relegate all the incurable diseases, or all the diseases the remedy for which they overlook, to witchcraft. When they do this, they are talking about disease as a blind man talks about colour.'

The following passage from G. B. Harrison's introduction to the transcripts of the trials of Lancaster witches provides an example to the point: 'As the child's sickness continued, her urine was sent to Cambridge to Dr Barrow, who could find no disease unless it was the worms; and made out an appropriate medicine. Two days later further specimens and medicines were exchanged, but still without any result. The third time of sending Dr Barrow then

demanded whether there was any sorcery or witchcraft suspected.'
This way out must have been particularly attractive to court
physicians who often had to suffer cruel punishment for failing to
cure their mighty patient. Nevertheless it seems unlikely that many
of them were cynical tricksters. It seems more plausible to imagine
that most of them were prompted by an inextricable mixture of
conceit, bluff, self-deception and superstition.

The tone of the writings clearly suggests that the fear was
genuine. However, it would be a fatuous error to imagine that
witch hunts were some kind of 'psychotherapy' designed to
alleviate guilt feelings. On the contrary, it is reasonable to suppose
that taking part in the gruesome proceedings might have prompted
additional feelings of guilt which would be repressed from consciousness, and through still more projection provide a further
stimulus for ferocity. Ferocity, however, in no way excludes fear.
On the contrary, there is a wide measure of agreement among
psychiatrists that commonly there is a close causal connection
between a repression of feelings of guilt and delusions of persecution. So, we can see here another self-reinforcing mental mechanism
(a 'positive feedback') which has helped to produce the state of
mind thus described by Lucien Fèvre in the article quoted earlier:

> Devils, devils! They are everywhere. They haunt the most
> intelligent of men of the age in the daytime and at night. Devils
> which introduce themselves into the bodies of men and especially
> of women; in such great numbers that Bossuet wrote: 'I hold
> that witches could form any army equal to that of Xerxes, which
> was at least 180,000 men. For if, under the reign of Charles IX,
> they numbered 300,000 in France alone how many will there be
> in the other countries?'
>
> And after referring to Germany which was entirely engaged 'in
> building bonfires for them', Switzerland, which had depopulated
> whole villages in order to get rid of them and Lorraine, which
> 'shows travellers a thousand-thousand gibbets on which it strings
> them up', all 'teeming in the earth like worms in our gardens',
> he explodes, 'I should like them all to be put into one single
> body so that they could be burned all together in a single flame!'[32]

The Witch Mania must also have been stimulated by the impact
of the psychoses caused by syphilis: general paresis or *dementia
paralytica*, tabes, and cerebral syphilis. Here are a few quotations

from a well known modern textbook of psychiatry:[33]

> *Dementia paralytica* may be defined as an organic disease of the
> brain, of an inflammatory and degenerative nature, manifesting
> itself in progressive mental deterioration, and accompanied by
> certain definite physical signs . . . The disease is world-wide,
> although it is less common in tropical countries . . . *Dementia
> paralytica* usually manifests itself at any time from five to twenty
> years after infection . . . The average rate at which the disease
> develops varies between thirty and fifty years, but cases below
> thirty and above fifty are relatively infrequent. Males are more
> often affected than females, in the proportion of four to one, but
> this variation does not occur in cases of juvenile general paralysis,
> where the sexes seem to be equally affected . . . Remissions may
> occur at any time during the course of the disease which may
> come even to an apparent standstill.
>   The disease is commonly insidious in its development, and is
> characterised by episodes of strange behaviour, not at all in
> harmony with the previous character of the individual . . . All
> the aesthetic feelings become lost. The relatives and friends
> cannot understand the alteration in the patient's personality, but
> feel that he is utterly different from what he formerly was . . .
> During the progress of the disease the memory is progressively
> impaired, not only of recent events, but more remote ones . . .
> There is disorientation, particularly for time.
>   Grandiose delusions, which are in this disease of a bizarre
> type, are not so common as has been generally supposed.
> Indeed, in some cases, instead of a feeling of well-being and
> euphoria, a state of intense depression is present, even amoun-
> ting to stupor with mutism. The feature of the depression is the
> frequency with which absurd nihilistic ideas are expressed.
> Patients claim that they are dead, that their blood has ceased to
> circulate, that they have no pulse, that their bodies are utterly
> destroyed. The ideas of the depressive type are as fantastic and
> grotesque as those of the grandiose variety . . . any type of
> mental picture may appear – cases, for instance, in which
> hallucinations are prominent, cases showing alternating elation
> and depression and cases in whom persecutory delusions are in
> the forefront . . . the first evidence of a general paralytic process
> may be the occurrence of a convulsive seizure, but more usually
> these seizures occur during the course of the disease.

One can well imagine how people showing the derangements described above would be seen as 'possessed', or 'bewitched', or having relations with the devil, particularly as nothing was known about the causation. On the latter point, Henderson and Gillespie say:

> During the past century this disease has been investigated from many different aspects, and its identity has been well established on clinical, pathological and serological grounds. For many years it has been recognised that many of those who ultimately suffered from this disease had at one time contracted a syphilitic infection, but there were many competent observers who stated that the condition could occur quite independently of any syphilitic infection – for instance from head injury, alcoholism or an erratic mode of life. The theory of the syphilitic causation of this disease was at first based entirely on statistics, but after Krafft-Ebing had had the temerity to inoculate general paralytics with syphilitic virus without infecting them, the conception of the syphilitic origin of the disease was greatly strengthened. This theory soon received further support from a series of researches on the cerebro-spinal fluid, originated by Widal and Sicard, and carried on by many others until Wassermann demonstrated antibodies in the cerebro-spinal fluid and blood serum of those known to be suffering from syphilitic disease affecting the nervous system.
>
> In 1913 Noguchi and Moore announced that in 14 out of 70 cases of general paralysis they had been able to demonstrate the *Treponema pallidum* in the brain cortex. These findings have been confirmed by many other observers. It can thus be definitively stated: 'No syphilis, no paresis.' While this is so, it does not necessarily mean that syphilis invariably leads to an affection of the nervous system; it has been estimated that approximately only 2% of syphilitics ever develop general paralysis. Why it develops in one case and not in another has been constantly discussed, but we still do not know whether it is a matter of a special strain of the organism or of a specially susceptible nervous system.

The lack of regularity in the development of the disease would facilitate attributions to occult forces. The same applies to cerebral syphilis. According to Henderson and Gillespie:

In the early stages of his illness the patient may complain of a certain nervous uneasiness, may feel dull, changed, mixed up in the head and complain of difficulty in thinking. The emotional condition is variable; at one time the patient is excited, irritable and resistive, while at another time he may be depressed, anxious and easily frightened . . . The delirium which sets in is of the usual kind. It is a hallucinatory state with fear, and with great difficulty in comprehension and in attention. The patient is imperfectly oriented for time and place . . . It is estimated that in the absence of head injury, upwards of 90% of all cases of ocular palsy in adults are caused by syphilis or by brain tumour.

We can hardly be surprised at the inability of the physicians of those days to understand the connection between the infection and the late and irregular symptoms when we read that even nowadays an early diagnosis presents difficulties. According to Price's *Textbook of the Practice of Medicine*[34]

The dementia may at first be quite undetectable as such, because it appears under the deceptive guise of a neurasthenia, melancholia, or mania: only gradually does the intellectual impairment become manifest. In the beginning of general paralysis, which is seldom abrupt (though it may need a careful inquiry to verify the prodromal symptoms), 'functional' syndromes can be so 'typical' and organic changes so slight that the most expert psychiatrist is misled; only by physical and serological examinations can he avoid a blunder. A faint degradation of personality, a lapse in social refinements may be the first indication of what is wrong. Then memory for the events of yesterday and last week becomes less trustworthy, what seemed at first a trivial absence of mind becomes a serious incapacity, and yet the patient remains serene and outwardly indifferent to his lapses.

Tabes was likely to prompt accusations, as can be seen from the following quotation from Price:[35]

A certain number of patients with *tabes dorsalis* develop general paralysis at a later date; but mental symptoms of other kinds may also develop in tabetics who show neither the physical nor the mental symptoms of general paralysis. The commonest nonparalytical syndromes appearing in tabetics are, according to Otto Meyer, chronic hallucinatory paranoid states, depressive psychoses, circular psychoses, acute hallucinatory confusion, hallucinatory anxious states and various types of dementia. Kraepelin believes that there is a psychosis which is commoner than any other in tabes, and which has a course, symptomatology and outcome distinct from general paralysis. This psychosis consists in an acute hallucinatory excitement. The patient suddenly becomes fearful, agitated, hears distinct voices and is accused of numerous crimes. The onset is sudden and later in life and often at a later stage in the course of tabes than general paralysis is accustomed to appear. Memory, retention and orientation remain intact, and speech and writing do not present the specific disturbances seen in cases of general paralysis. The symptoms may subside in a few months, or remain indefinitely.

Given the ignorance of the causes, coupled with the unquestioned belief that Witchcraft can cause disease and possession, it would be strange if a spectacular eruption of the derangements described above did not foster the notion that witches were proliferating and intensifying their nefarious activities.

Moreover, these diseases multiplied the number of people whose strange behaviour aroused suspicions, as well as the number of paranoiacs eager to issue accusations. The ratio of male to female sufferers from these psychoses is 4 to 1, according to Henderson and Gillespie, which would fuel the tendency to demonise women. It may not be a coincidence that this is a rough converse of the sex ratio among the victims of the trials, as estimated by Delumeau. Persecutory hallucinations, caused by syphilitic psychoses, may have prompted much of the preaching and theorising about Witches and Satan. This might have been the case with Jean Bodin.

Although neurotic difficulties connected with his celibacy might have had something to do with it, Isaac Newton's acceptance of the current beliefs about witches might be explained as partly due to the intensity of his preoccupation with mathematical theories; this did not leave him enough mental energy for a critical examination of matters unrelated to his studies, so that his writings about witches were a kind of self-indulgence. In contrast, Jean Bodin (1530–96) was perhaps the greatest innovator in the study of society between Macchiavelli and Montesquieu; he was not generally inclined to receive uncritically the current opinions about human behaviour, and was well acquainted with good arguments to the contrary. Indeed, one of his two works on Witchcraft was a polemic against Johannes Weyer – a brave author who criticised the current beliefs about witches on good grounds of commonsense logic. What is even more incongruous, Bodin wrote a work called *Heptalomeres*, which he kept hidden during his life and which was only published in 1914; there he advocates the equality of religions before the law and appears to be an agnostic. Yet at the age of forty-eight he wrote his bloodthirsty treatise on witches; after that he wrote only a book on nature which is regarded by later commentators as showing a conspicuous decline of his mental powers.

Bodin writes about witches making men impotent. The treatise was printed two years after his marriage at forty-six. (Of his three children, one died early, another was mentally defective, and the third insane.) According to some of his biographers he remained a bachelor until then, including during his years at the licentious French court, while others say that he was a defrocked Carmelite monk who had earlier married and divorced a woman of ill repute. In either case he had a good chance of contracting syphilis. The difference in quality between his earlier and later works indicates a deterioration of the brain which cannot be attributed to normal senility as he died at the age of 66. The man who adumbrated the quantity theory of money and who could see (contrary to the universally held belief) that gold does not constitute real wealth, would not accept the plain logic of Weyer's arguments: e.g. that if the witches were so powerful that they could do all the things attributed to them, then surely they would also be able to escape from prison or avoid arrest. Bodin's fulminations also show the common feature of neurotic and psychotic obsessions; namely, the exclusion of any possibility of a refutation by the facts. He insists that evidence which in other matters would be sufficient for a verdict of 'not guilty', must not be accepted in witch trials. His views on this matter were generally followed.

The general inclination of all pre-scientific cultures to attribute disease to witchcraft was often strengthened by the fusion of the functions of the priest and the healer. According to Andrew D. White,

Especially prejudicial to a true development of medical science among the first Christians was their attribution of disease to diabolic influence. As we have seen, this idea had come from far, and, having prevailed in Chaldea, Egypt, and Persia, had naturally entered into the sacred books of the Hebrews. Moreover, St Paul had distinctly declared that the gods of the heathen were devils; and everywhere the early Christians saw in disease the malignant work of these dethroned powers of evil. The Gnostic and Manichæan struggles had ripened the theologic idea that, although at times diseases are punishments by the Almighty, the main agency in them is Satanic. The great fathers and renowned leaders of the early Church accepted and strengthened this idea. Origen said: 'It is demons which produce famine, unfruitfulness, corruptions of the air, pestilences; they hover concealed in clouds in the lower atmosphere, and are attracted by the blood and incense which the heathen offer to them as gods.' St Augustine said: 'All diseases of Christians are to be ascribed to these demons; chiefly do they torment fresh-baptized Christians, yea, even the guiltless, newborn infants.' Tertullian insisted that a malevolent angel is in constant attendance upon every person. Gregory of Nazianzus declared that bodily pains are provoked by demons, and that medicines are useless, but that they are often cured by the laying on of consecrated hands. St Nilus and St Gregory of Tours, echoing St Ambrose, gave examples to show the sinfulness of resorting to medicine instead of trusting to the intercession of saints.

St Bernard, in a letter to certain monks, warned them that to seek relief from disease in medicine was in harmony neither with their religion nor with the honour and purity of their order. This view even found its way into the canon law, which declared the precepts of medicine contrary to Divine knowledge. As a rule, the leaders of the Church discouraged the theory that diseases are due to natural causes, and most of them deprecated a resort to surgeons and physicians rather than to supernatural means.

Out of these and similar considerations was developed the vast system of 'pastoral medicine,' so powerful not only through the Middle Ages, but even in modern times, both among Catholics and Protestants. As to its results, we must bear in mind that, while there is no need to attribute the mass of stories regarding miraculous cures to conscious fraud, there was without doubt, at a later period, no small admixture of belief biased by self-interest, with much pious invention and suppression of facts. Enormous revenues flowed into various monasteries and churches in all parts of Europe from relics noted for their healing powers. Every cathedral, every great abbey, and nearly every parish church claimed possession of healing relics. While, undoubtedly, a childlike faith was at the bottom of this belief, there came out of it unquestionably a great development of the mercantile spirit. The commercial value of sundry relics was often very high. In the year 1056 a French ruler pledged securities to the amount of ten thousand solidi for the production of the relics of St Just and St Pastor, pending a legal decision regarding the ownership between him and the Archbishop of Narbonne. The Emperor of Germany on one occasion demanded, as a sufficient pledge for the establishment of a city market, the arm of St George. The body of St Sebastian brought enormous wealth to the Abbey of Soissons; Rome, Canterbury, Treves, Marburg, every great city, drew large revenues from similar sources and the Venetian Republic ventured very considerable sums in the purchase of relics.

Naturally, then, corporations, whether lay or ecclesiastical, which drew large revenue from relics looked with little favour on a science which tended to discredit their investments . . .;

We find cropping out everywhere the feeling that, since supernatural means are so abundant, there is something irreligious in seeking cure by natural means; ever and anon we have appeals to Scripture, and especially to the case of King Asa, who trusted to physicians rather than to the priests of Jahveh, and so died. Hence it was that St Bernard declared that monks who took medicine were guilty of conduct unbecoming to religion. Even the School of Salerno was held in aversion by multitudes of strict churchmen, since it prescribed rules for diet, thereby indicating a belief that diseases arise from natural causes and not from the malice of the devil: moreover, in the medical schools Hippocrates was studied, and he had especially declared that demoniacal possession is 'nowise more divine nowise more infernal, than any other disease.' Hence it was, doubtless, that the Lateran Council, about the beginning of the thirteenth century, forbade physicians, under pain of exclusion from the Church, to undertake medical treatment without calling in ecclesiastical advice. . . .

This view was long cherished in the Church, and nearly two

hundred and fifty years later Pope Pius V revived it by renewing the command of Pope Innocent and enforcing it with penalties. Not only did Pope Pius order that all physicians before administering treatment should call in 'a physician of the soul,' on the ground, as he declares, that 'bodily infirmity frequently arises from sin,' but he ordered that, if at the end of three days the patient had not made confession to a priest, the medical man should cease his treatment, under pain of being deprived of his right to practise, and of expulsion from the faculty if he were a professor, and that every physician and professor of medicine should make oath that he was strictly fulfilling these conditions.[36]

Given the desire of the Churches to supply and monopolise medical care (to use today's words), their inability to stop the spread of the disease might sow doubt about its teaching and even undermine the loyalty of the flock. By attributing the ills to an increased activity of Satan and a proliferation of witches, the Churchmen not only staved off doubt and defection but actually raised the demand for their services and the dependence of the flock on them. The way of thinking is vividly depicted in the following quotation from White:

> But this sort of theological reasoning developed an idea . . . that Satan, in causing pestilences, used as his emissaries especially Jews and witches. The proof of this belief in the case of the Jews was seen in the fact that they escaped with a less percentage of disease than did the Christians in the great plague periods. This was doubtless due in some measure to their remarkable sanitary system, which had probably originated thousands of years before in Egypt, and had been handed down through Jewish lawgivers and statesmen. Certainly they observed more careful sanitary rules and more constant abstinence from dangerous foods than was usual among Christians; but the public at large could not understand so simple a cause, and jumped to the conclusion that their immunity resulted from protection by Satan, and that this protection was repaid and the pestilence caused by their wholesale poisoning of Christians. As a result of this mode of thought, attempts were made in all parts of Europe to propitiate the Almighty, to thwart Satan, and to stop the plague by torturing and murdering the Jews. Throughout Europe during great pestilences we hear of extensive burnings of this devoted people. In Bavaria, at the time of the Black

Death, it is computed that twelve thousand Jews thus perished; in the small town of Erfurt the number is said to have been three thousand; in Strasburg, the Rue Brulée remains as a monument to the two thousand Jews burned there for poisoning the wells and causing the plague of 1348; at the royal castle of Chinon, near Tours, an immense trench was dug, filled with blazing wood, and in a single day one hundred and sixty Jews were burned. Everywhere in continental Europe this mad persecution went on; but it is a pleasure to say that one great churchman, Pope Clement VI, stood against this popular unreason and, so far as he could bring his influence to bear on the maddened populace, exercised it in favour of mercy to these supposed enemies of the Almighty.[37]

The Churchmen's hostility to anything smacking of a naturalistic approach to diseases was strengthened by the fact that the chief exponents of this view were to be found among the infidels. As White says,

From a very early period of European history the Jews had taken the lead in medicine; their share in founding the great schools of Salerno and Montpellier we have already noted, and in all parts of Europe we find them acknowledged leaders in the healing art. The Church authorities, enforcing the spirit of the time, were especially severe against these benefactors: that men who openly rejected the means of salvation, and whose souls were undeniably lost, should heal the elect seemed an insult to Providence: preaching friars denounced them from the pulpit, and the rulers in state and church, while frequently secretly consulting them, openly proscribed them.

Gregory of Tours tells us of an archdeacon who, having been partially cured of disease of the eyes by St Martin, sought further aid from a Jewish physician, with the result that neither the saint nor the Jew could help him afterward. Popes Eugene IV, Nicholas V, and Calixtus III especially forbade Christians to employ them. The Trullanean Council in the eighth century, the Councils of Béziers and Alby in the thirteenth, the Councils of Avignon and Salamanca in the fourteenth, the Synod of Bamberg and the Bishop of Passau in the fifteenth, the Council of Avignon in the sixteenth, with many others, expressly forbade the faithful to call Jewish physicians or surgeons; such great preachers as

John Geiler and John Herolt thundered from the pulpit against them and all who consulted them. As late as the middle of the seventeenth century, when the City Council of Hall, in Würtemberg, gave some privileges to a Jewish physician 'on account of his admirable experience and skill,' the clergy of the city joined in a protest, declaring that 'it were better to die with Christ than to be cured by a Jew doctor aided by the devil.' Still, in their extremity, bishops, cardinals, kings, and even popes, insisted on calling in physcians of the hated race.

The Reformation made no sudden change in the sacred theory of medicine. Luther, as is well known, again and again ascribed his own diseases to 'devils' spells,' declaring that 'Satan produces all the maladies which afflict mankind, for he is the prince of death,' and that 'he poisons the air'; but that 'no malady comes from God.' From that day down to the faith cures of Boston, Old Orchard, and among the sect of 'Peculiar People' in our own time, we see the results among Protestants of seeking the cause of disease in Satanic influence and its cure in fetichism.[38]

Even today psychiatry remains the least effective branch of medicine and the most open to quackery. The situation at the time of the Witch Craze is described in the following quotations from White:

If ordinary diseases were likely to be attributed to diabolical agency, how much more diseases of the brain, and especially the more obscure of these! These, indeed, seemed to the vast majority of mankind possible only on the theory of Satanic intervention: any approach to a true theory of the connection between physical causes and mental results is one of the highest acquisitions of science.

Here and there, during the whole historic period, keen men had obtained an inkling of the truth; but to the vast multitude, down to the end of the seventeenth century, nothing was more clear than that insanity is, in many if not in most cases, demoniacal possession.

The first main weapon against the indwelling Satan continued to be the exorcism; but under the influence of inferences from Scripture farther and farther fetched, and of theological reasoning more and more subtle, it became something very different from the gentle procedure of earlier times, and some description of this great weapon at the time of its highest development will throw light on the laws which govern the growth of theological reasoning, as well as upon the main subject in hand.

A fundamental premise in the fully developed exorcism was that, according to sacred Scripture, a main characteristic of Satan is pride. Pride led him to rebel; for pride he was cast down; therefore the first thing to do, in driving him out of a lunatic, was to strike a fatal blow at his pride – to disgust him.

This theory was carried out logically, to the letter. The treatises on the subject simply astound one by their wealth of blasphemous and obscene epithets which it was allowable for the exorcist to use in casting out devils. The *Treasury of Exorcisms* contains hundreds of pages packed with the vilest epithets which the worst imagination could invent for the purpose of overwhelming the indwelling Satan.

Some of those decent enough to be printed in these degenerate days ran as follows:

'Thou lustful and stupid one, . . . thou lean sow, famine-stricken and most impure, . . . thou wrinkled beast, thou mangy beast, thou beast of all beasts the most beastly, . . . thou mad spirit, . . . thou bestial and foolish drunkard, . . . most greedy wolf, . . . most abominable whisperer, . . . thou sooty spirit from Tartarus! . . . I cast thee down, O Tartarean boor, into the infernal kitchen! . . . Loathsome cobbler, . . . dingy collier, . . . filthy sow (*scrofa stercorata*), . . . perfidious boar, . . . envious crocodile, . . . malodorous drudge, . . . wounded basilisk, . . . rust-coloured asp, . . . swollen toad, . . . entangled spider, . . . lousy swineherd (*porcarie pedicose*), . . . lowest of the low, . . . cudgelled ass,' etc.

But, in addition to this attempt to disgust Satan's pride with blackguardism, there was another to scare him with tremendous words. For this purpose, thunderous names, from Hebrew and Greek, were imported, such as Acharon, Eheye, Schemhamphora, Tetragrammaton, Homöousion, Athanatos, Ischiros, Æcodes, and the like.

Efforts were also made to drive him out with filthy and rank-smelling drugs; and, among those which can be mentioned in a printed article, we may name asafœtida, sulphur, squills, etc., which were to be burned under his nose.

Still further to plague him, pictures of the devil were to be spat upon, trampled under foot by people of low condition, and sprinkled with foul compounds. . . . Vast numbers were punished as tabernacles of Satan.

One of the least terrible of these punishments, and perhaps the most common of all, was that of scourging demons out of the body of a lunatic. This method commended itself even to the judgment of so thoughtful and kindly a personage as Sir Thomas More, and as late as the sixteenth century. But if the disease continued, as it naturally would after such treatment, the authorities frequently felt justified in driving out the demons by torture.

Interesting monuments of this idea, so fruitful in evil, still exist. In the great cities of central Europe, 'witch towers,' where witches and demoniacs were tortured, and 'fool towers,' where the more gentle lunatics were imprisoned, may still be seen.

In the cathedrals we still see this idea fossilized. Devils and imps, struck into stone, clamber upon towers, prowl under cornices, peer out from bosses of foliage, perch upon capitals, nestle under benches, flame in windows. Above the great main entrance, the most common of all representations still shows Satan and his imps scowling, jeering, grinning, while taking possession of the souls of men and scourging them with serpents, or driving them with tridents, or dragging them with chains into the flaming mouth of hell. Even in the most hidden and sacred places of the mediæval cathedral we still find representations of Satanic power in which profanity and obscenity run riot. In these representations the painter and the glass-stainer vied with the sculptor. Among the early paintings on canvas a well-known example represents the devil in the shape of a dragon, perched near the head of a dying man, eager to seize his soul as it issues from his mouth, and only kept off by the efforts of the attendant priest. Typical are the colossal portrait of Satan, and the vivid picture of the devils cast out of the possessed and entering into the swine, as shown in the cathedral-windows of Strasburg. So, too, in the windows of Chartres Cathedral we see a saint healing a lunatic: the saint, with a long devil-scaring formula in Latin issuing from his mouth; and the lunatic with a little detestable hobgoblin, horned, hoofed, and tailed, issuing from *his* mouth. These examples are but typical of myriads in cathedrals and abbeys and parish churches throughout Europe; and all served to impress upon the popular mind a horror of everything called diabolic, and a hatred of those charged with it. These sermons in stones preceded the printed book; they were a sculptured Bible, which preceded Luther's pictorial Bible.

The reformed Church in all its branches fully accepted the doctrines of witchcraft and diabolic possession, and developed them still further. No one urged their fundamental ideas more fully than Luther. He did, indeed, reject portions of the witchcraft folly; but to the influence of devils he not only attributed his maladies, but his dreams, and nearly everything that thwarted or disturbed him. The flies which lighted upon his book, the rats which kept him awake at night, he believed to be devils; the resistance of the Archbishop of Mayence to his ideas, he attributed to Satan literally working in that prelate's heart; to his disciples he told stories of men who had been killed by rashly resisting the devil. Insanity, he was quite sure, was caused by Satan, and he exorcised sufferers. Against some he appears to have advised stronger remedies; and his horror of idiocy, as resulting from Satanic influence, was so great, that on one occasion he appears to have advised the killing of an idiot child, as being the direct offspring of Satan. Yet Luther was one of the most tender and loving of men; in the whole range of literature there is hardly anything more touching than his words and tributes to children. In enforcing his ideas regarding insanity, he laid stress especially upon the question of St Paul as to the bewitching of the Galatians, and, regarding idiocy, on the account in Genesis of the birth of children whose fathers were 'sons of God' and whose mothers were 'daughters of men.'

One idea of his was especially characteristic. The descent of Christ into hell was a frequent topic of discussion in the Reformed Church. Melanchthon, with his love of Greek studies, held that the purpose of the Saviour in making such a descent was to make himself known to the great and noble men of antiquity – Plato, Socrates, and the rest; but Luther insisted that his purpose was to conquer Satan in a hand-to-hand struggle.

This idea of diabolic influence pervaded his conversation, his preaching, his writings, and spread thence to the Lutheran Church in general.

Calvin also held to the same theory, and having more power with less kindness of heart than Luther, carried it out with yet greater harshness. Beza was especially severe against those who believed insanity to be a natural malady, and declared, 'Such persons are refuted both by sacred and profane history.'

Under the influence, then, of such infallible teachings, in the older Church and in the new, this superstition was developed more and more into cruelty; and as the biblical texts, popularized in the sculptures and windows and mural decorations of the great mediæval cathedrals, had done much to develop it among the people, so Luther's translation of the Bible, especially in the numerous editions of it illustrated with engravings, wrought with enormous power to spread and deepen it. In every peasant's cottage some one could spell out the story of the devil bearing Christ through the air and placing him upon the pinnacle of the Temple – of the woman with seven devils – of the devils cast into the swine. Every peasant's child could be made to understand the quaint pictures in the family Bible or the catechism which illustrated vividly all those texts.[39]

Treatment with mercury – the only therapy which had real, as opposed to purely imaginary effects, and could attenuate and up to a point contain the progress of the disease – provided an additional stimulus to the spread of the craze. Even well before the end of the seventeenth century most physicians knew that very big doses of mercury will make patients ill or might even kill them. But only in recent times has it been discovered that prolonged absorption of even very small doses can seriously damage the central nervous system. According to Price's *Textbook of the Practice of Medicine*:

Ingestion of the corrosive salt is followed at once by burning pain, blood-stained vomiting, and diarrhoea. The mouth becomes red and sore and the mucosa ulcerates. There is a strong metallic taste. There is a continuous flux and much pain from the bowels for several days. Oliguria is inevitable and the chief danger to life lies in renal or hepatic failure, but complete recovery is possible. Subacute or chronic poisoning such as follows contamination of a food source may affect the central nervous system, giving rise to erethism, tremors and degenerative lesions. Excessive salivation, foetor and a blue line on the gums occur. The alkyl mercurials in particular cause nervous symptoms. Blindness and paresis are permanent. Rare forms of mercurialism include dermatosis in adults, aerodynia in infants, granulocylopenia, and opacity of the optic lens.

Symptoms: The symptoms of mercury poisoning include

tremor, erethism, gingivitis, stomatitis, mercurialentis, and skin disorders. The tremor is quite distinctive as can be seen from the phrases 'hatter's shakes' or 'Danbury shakes' (Danbury is a suburb of New York where there used to be many hat factories). It can be demonstrated by asking the patient to write his name or make a drawing. The tremor affects not only the hands but the corners of the mouth, the tongue and face and later the arms, feet, and legs.

Erethism is a condition peculiar to mercury poisoning. It consists of an abnormal shyness with all the attendant signs of blushing, stammering, timidity, indecision, overreaction to criticism, and even frank weeping. It is this condition which led to the phrase 'as mad as a hatter'. Further effects on the nervous system may involve ataxia, spasticity, and loss of sensation to such a degree as to be mistaken for multiple sclerosis.[40]

Like cerebral syphilis, mercury poisoning must have reinforced the obsessive fear of witches by producing a crop of sufferings which would be interpreted as signs of bewitchment. Secondly, it caused a multiplication of individuals with impaired brains who were particularly prone to gullibility and delusions, and therefore, predisposed towards launching or backing accusations. This might have been the case with King James I who constantly urinated in his pants, exuded an unpleasant smell and received various kinds of medication.

By taking into consideration the medical factor one can also explain why the Witch Craze affected Spain and Italy less than the countries to the north, and southern Italy less than northern. In 1917 J. Wagner-Jauregg in Vienna began to treat patients suffering from cerebral syphilis by infecting them with malaria, and until the discovery of penicillin this was the only effective cure. Naturally-acquired malaria has the same effect. Henderson and Gillespie report that syphilitic psychoses are rare in the tropics; nowadays malaria is rare outside tropical zones. In the earlier centuries, however, it was common in the southern parts of Europe. Consequently, the impact of syphilis could not have had there the same devastating force which it had further north. In addition to the cultural factors mentioned earlier, malaria may also have impeded the spread of the Witch Craze to the Balkans.

It remains to be added that, owing to the unfreedom of women, the ruling élites of the Islamic states should not have suffered from syphilis as much as their Christian equivalents. All important Moslem men had harems, guarded by eunuchs, containing women recruited as virgins and well inspected beforehand. Such men had little incentive for adultery or brothel-crawling, and their wives and concubines had no opportunities for straying. Consequently, the Moslem magnates were unlikely to catch venereal disease, which was rife among the nobility and royalty of Europe, actually caused the dying out of a number of dynasties, and must have contributed to the bizarre behaviour of monarchs like Henry VIII and Ivan the Terrible.

In contrast to the historical processes invoked in other explanations, the epidemic of syphilis shows a perfect chronological correspondence with the Witch Craze. Trials, which were sporadic during the preceding centuries, multiplied enormously after 1500 and at the same time the sex ratio among the victims swung drastically against women. The epidemic of syphilis struck a few years earlier. Witch hunting petered out gradually and at different times in various parts of Europe during the second half of the seventeenth century, and ceased altogether during the eighteenth. This was also the time when syphilis began to assume somewhat milder forms. According to W. H. McNeill's study of plagues:

> By the end of the [16th] century, syphilis began to recede. The more fulminant forms of infection were dying out, as the normal sorts of adjustment between host and parasite asserted themselves, i.e. as milder strains of the spirochete displaced those that killed off their hosts too rapidly, and as the resistance of European populations to the organism increased.[41]

As the historian of medicine Charles Singer says, considerable progress was made around 1700 in the treatment:[42]

> Its treatment by mercury had been practised at least as early as the fifteenth century, perhaps as an inheritance from the Arabic-speaking physicians. During the sixteenth and seventeenth centuries various other remedies were tried; much quackery arose around them. In the eighteenth century the accumulated experience of generations returned again to mercury. Satisfactory

methods of administration were evolved and the treatment
became standardized. It hardly changed until the twentieth
century.

Development of the disease became as a rule slower, and its most
vivid manifestations (like the rotting away of the flesh) came later
and more rarely.

The fact that the craze spread quickly and petered out slowly
and unevenly – which is a sequence normally encountered in
epidemics to which the ravages of syphilis in the sixteenth and
seventeenth centuries has conformed – constitutes another argument for linking the two phenomena.

According to some historians a certain abatement (though by no
means a cessation) of the persecutions had occurred between 1530
and 1560 or 1580. This cannot be explained with assurance on
medico-psychoanalytic lines without a deeper study of the social
history of the epidemic. There is some evidence that virulence of
the disease had slightly subsided during this period but much
more research is needed to substantiate this view. However, even
if there were good reasons for assuming that there has been no
such respite, the general thesis would not be invalidated because
it would be surprising if there was a simple linear relationship
between the epidemic and the intensity of the reaction to it. Social
processes are so complex, fluid and without clear boundaries, that
it is not surprising that very few (if any) connections between them
can be adequately described by linear equations, particularly as
the delays between the precipitant and the reactions to it often
display apparently random variations. However, although the
aforesaid abatement can be reconciled with an epidemiological
explanation, it does invalidate explanations in terms of the inertia
of beliefs or institutions, which must be assumed to have been
constant if such explanations are to have any sense at all.

In passing I must say a few words in defence of the thesis against
a possible objection on the ground that if syphilis were the chief
cause of the obsessive fear of witches, then the persecutions should
have occurred mainly in the seaports and big cities, whereas some
of the bloodiest hunts took place in remote mountainous regions.
The first part of the answer is that this statement is not entirely
correct: it is true that some seaports (London and Amsterdam)
witnessed relatively few trials, but others (for example Bordeaux
and Rouen) were scenes of massive persecutions. Secondly, the

mountainous regions (especially of Switzerland) supplied a disproportionate number of mercenaries to all European armies who of
all men were the most likely to catch the disease, which they would
bring back to their villages. Such regions might be even more
severely afflicted than the seaports because sailors had much less
opportunity for fornication and rape, while they were much more
likely to get malaria.

Presumably under the influence of the modern superstition that
everything must have an economic cause, the historians failed to
investigate the connection of the Witch Craze with disease and
celibacy, although clear clues were furnished long ago by the
Victorian historian William H. Lecky. In the chapter on witchcraft
in the first volume of his *Rise and Development of Rationalism in
Europe*,[43] Lecky talks about the advances of celibacy through the
proliferation of the monastic orders and about the shock of the
plague – The Black Death. He seems to regard the plague as the
more fundamental factor, suggesting that the multiplication of the
monasteries and nunneries, as well as the spread of fanatical
movements like the Flagellants, were reactions to the shock of the
disease which made people feel that the world is a vale of tears.
Lecky does not mention syphilis, presumably because he did not
know its history.

Although he makes it clear that he feels that there is a connection,
Lecky is not very specific about its nature. Writing several decades
before Freud, he could not have analysed the mental mechanism
in the way I have done here, which makes it all the more remarkable
that he saw the connection. Furthermore, even if he had known
about the history of syphilis, Lecky might not have thought of it
as the main precipitant of the persecutions because he dated the
flaring up thereof from the beginning of the fifteenth century
instead of from its end, as today's historians do. Given the
advantage of a century of research, the latter must be right about
the dating of the biggest wave but a minor intensification seems
to have occurred as Lecky said, and he probably is right about
attributing the advance of celibacy to the effects of the Black Death.

With the help of the psychoanalytic concepts of the censor,
repression, projection of desire, aggression and guilt, ambivalence
and inversion of desire into hate and scapegoating; knowing about
the frustration-aggression mechanism and the aetiology of paranoid
states, we can make a much better case than Lecky does for linking
celibacy, puritanism, disease and the obsession about witches.

The medical interpretation accounts also for some other coincidences noted by historians, which up till now have appeared completely mysterious. In his studies of the persecutions in Germany, H. C. Erik Midelfort[44] maintains that the regions where these were the most severe were distinguished by an unusually high ratio of single women. This connection becomes explicable when we bear in mind that such a ratio would encourage fornication and, therefore, increase contagion and panic. We can also account for the numerous instances of witch hunts following in the wake of military campaigns – which led many historians as we saw earlier to follow a wrong track in the search for an explanation. The link is clear: soldiers have always been the most effective spreaders of venereal disease, particularly in the epoch when they regarded rape as their natural right. The special victimisation of midwives, noted in most histories of the persecutions, also ceases to be inexplicable: during the epidemic the number of stillbirths, infantile deaths, and children born with deformations must have increased dramatically; and midwives would be the obvious scapegoats.

It is possible that some of the witches execrated as 'ugly' were syphilitic; some might have been in fact agents of contagion. Nor should we assume that all the women described as 'old' must have been sexually inactive; in those days every woman over thirty would be called old. Among the tormentors' prurient sadistic enjoyments was the practice of poking the victims with their fingers all over the naked body in search of insensitive spots which were regarded as a proof of being a witch. As syphilitics do, in fact, develop insensitive spots, this practice constitutes another pointer to the connection between the persecutions and the disease.

It is also possible that some of the accused were retired prostitutes. It would, however, be a gross error to imagine that the Witch Hunts might have been some rational method of extirpating the carriers of the disease. Once the fear and hatred of women became widespread, the choice of scapegoats would become quite random or determined by circumstances which had nothing to do with the danger of contagion. After the outbreaks of bubonic plague or cholera, we know that the mobs did not pick on soldiers but on Jews, or Gipsies, or some other defenceless minority.

Apart from accounting for the already mentioned characteristics of the craze, my thesis – unlike other interpretations – also explains its classless character as well as the intellectual current which accompanied the persecutions. If the craze was a mere parish-pump affair (as Thomas and Macfarlane try to tell us), why did prestigious authorities (including King James I) write books calling for general persecutions? On the other hand, if it was a clearly repressive action against the common folk organised by the ruling class (as Favret and, to some extent, Mandrou see it), then why did so many ordinary people launch the accusations, ask the authorities for help in finding witches, and even proceed to lynch the suspects? If it was a by-product of the functioning of the Church's repressive machinery, then why did so many authors write about witches? And why did their books find so many buyers, even when the authors were Catholic and the readers were Protestant? There is no way in which the demand for the English editions of the *Malleus* in the seventeenth century could be explained by the momentum of the Papal Inquisition. Such an explanation would not be valid even for a Catholic land. In modern totalitarian states, writings of the rulers and their propagandists can be distributed in large numbers to bookshops and libraries although not a soul wants to buy or read them. In the sixteenth and the seventeenth centuries, however, printing and bookselling was a small business wholly dependent on private buyers. The literature therefore provides a reliable indication of the state of mind of the literate classes.

My thesis, like a weather map, can account only for broad trends and conditions, and leaves out of consideration the local variations which may have been due to chance factors such as the character of individuals in crucial social or political positions. Still, detailed research into primary sources from the proffered viewpoint might also reveal closer covariation between the epidemic and the intensity of persecutions, and thus account for local differences.

As it stands, my thesis explains the following features of the great Witch Craze which up till now have appeared as inexplicable: (1) its duration; (2) the geographical extension; (3) its generality and classlessness; (4) its bias against women; (5) its contrariety to the direction of the intellectual progress occurring at the time; (6) its bias against midwives; (7) its loose association with wars; (8) the prominent role of monks and Puritans in the hounding and the greater ferocity of the former. I hope that the foregoing comparative analysis will stimulate research into primary sources which will throw more light on the interplay of the factors surveyed here.

Let me recapitulate. The underlying permanent condition was the prevalence of the belief that Witchcraft works and can cause disease. One of the preparatory conditions was the existence of the machinery of repression forged against heretics by the Church. The second preparatory condition was the demonisation of women, which was an exacerbation of an old ingredient of the Christian tradition, and a consequence of the tightening up of celibacy. The precipitating factor was the arrival of syphilis at the beginning of the sixteenth century which evoked panic and a search for scapegoats, chosen with preference from among the most defenceless members of the subjugated sex. A host of inexplicable psychoses and congenital malformations provided an additional stimulus for Witch Hunts. During the closing decades of the seventeenth century, and to an even great extent during the early part of the eighteenth, there was an abatement of the severity of the disease. This, together with the growing influence of a more advanced body of scientific knowledge and the decline of the influence of celibate clergy, led to the disappearance of the mania among Europe's educated classes, which brought the trials to an historic end.

Notes

1. S. Andreski, *Max Weber's Insights and Errors* (London: Routledge and Kegan Paul, 1982).
2. H. R. Trevor-Roper, *Religion, the Reformation and Social Change* (London: Macmillan, 1967) pp. 92–3.
3. Claudia Honegger, *Die Hexen der Neuzeit* (Frankfurt: Suhrkamp Verlag, 1978).
4. Jean Delumeau, *La Peur en Occident* (Paris: Librairie Arthème Fayard, 1978).
5. Keith Thomas, *Religion and the Decline of Magic* (London, 1971).
6. A survey of these and other estimates can be found in Delumeau, op. cit., p. 456.
7. Wilhelm Gottlieb Soldan, *Geschichte der Hexenprozesse: Aus den Quellen dargestellt* (Stuttgart, 1843; neu hrsg. von Heinrich Heppe, 2 Bde, Stuttgart, 1880; neu bearb, von Max Bauer, 2 Bde, München, 1912).
8. As summarised in Delumeau, op. cit.
9. E. William Monter, 'Witchcraft in Geneva', *Journal of Modern History*, 43, 1971.
10. Jeanne Favret, 'Sorcières et Lumières', in: *Critique*, 27, 1971.
11. Kurt Baschwitz, *Hexen und Hexenprozesse* (München: Deutscher Taschenbuch); Robert Mandrou, *Magistrates et sorciers en France au XVIIᵉ siècle. Une analyse de psychologie historique* (Paris, 1968).

12. Lucien Fèvre, *A New Kind of History*, ed. Peter Burke, transl. K. Folca (London: Routledge and Kegan Paul, 1973) p. 188.
13. Montague Summers, *The Geography of Witchcraft* (London: Kegan Paul, Trech Trubner & Co., 1927) p. 238.
14. Alan Macfarlane, *Witchcraft in Tudor and Stuart England* (London, 1970).
15. Mandrou, op. cit.
16. Trevor-Roper, op. cit., Chap. 3, 'The European Witch-craze of the Sixteenth and Seventeenth Centuries.'
17. Baschwitz, op. cit.
18. Soldan, op. cit.
19. Margaret Murray, *The Witch-Cult in Western Europe. A Study in Anthropology* (London: 1921).
20. As quoted in Baschwitz, op. cit.
21. Summers, op. cit., p. 65.
22. The statements about the baths are based on a personal communication from Prof. George Lehman.
23. Sigmund Freud, 'Eine Teufelsneurose im siebzehnten Jahrhundert', in *Gesammelte Werken, 13* (London, 1950).
24. See H. E. Feine, *Kirchliche Rechtsgeschichte* (Hermann Bohlaus Nachfolger, 1954).
25. Henry C. Lea, *History of Sacerdotal Celibacy in the Christian Church* (London: Watts & Co., 1932) pp. 299–300.
26. A Spanish physician claims that the students at theological seminaries have less developed pubic hair than other students. This suggests that nowadays they are self-selected for a weak sexual appetite. There is no reason to suppose that this was the case when priesthood was the only channel of social ascent for the poor and the dumping ground for disinherited younger sons of the aristocracy. See Gregorio Marañon, *Tres estudios sobre la vida sexual* (Madrid (no date)).
27. As quoted in Baschwitz, op. cit. The translation is mine.
28. As quoted in Delumeau, op. cit.
29. Jacobus Sprenger and Heinrich Krämer, *Malleus Maleficarum* (London: The Folio Society, 1968) pp. 29, 18–19, 51, 172, 176, 75, 71, 77, 80, 80–1, 45, 76, 177, 83, 87, 90–1, 93, 42, 44, 44.
30. As quoted by Delumeau, op. cit., p. 289. The translation is mine.
31. Summers, op. cit., p. 116.
32. Fèvre, op. cit.
33. Henderson and Gillespie, *A Text-Book of Psychiatry for Students and Practitioners* (London: Oxford University Press, 1950) pp. 466–9, 464–5, 493–5, 497.
34. Price, *Textbook of the Practice of Medicine*, 12th edn (Oxford, 1978) p. 1422.
35. Ibid.
36. Andrew D. White, *A History of the Warfare of Science with Theology*, vol. II (London: Arco Publishers, 1955) pp. 27–9, 37.
37. Ibid., p. 73.
38. Ibid., pp. 45–6.
39. Ibid., pp. 98, 106–7, 114–5.
40. Price, op. cit., pp. 271, 280.

41. W. H. McNeill, *Plagues and People* (Oxford: Basil Blackwell, 1976) p. 220.
42. Charles Singer, *A Short History of Medicine* (Oxford: Clarendon Press, 1928) p. 162.
43. Lecky, *The Rise and Development of Rationalism in Europe*, Vol. I.
44. H. C. Erik Midelfort, *Witch Hunting in South-Western Germany, 1582–1684* (Stanford, 1972).

Part Two
The Demonologists' Fascination with Lust and Disease illustrated from the Sources

QUEVERDO and DÜRER

These paintings show that (in contrast to the notion spread by more recent story books) Dürer did not have the image of a witch as beyond the age of sexual activity, while Queverdo imagined them as extremely attractive.

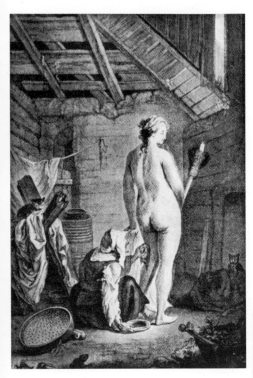

Queverdo: Off to the Sabbat.
Source: Montague Summers, *History of Witchcraft and Demonology,* Routledge and Kegan Paul, London: 1926.

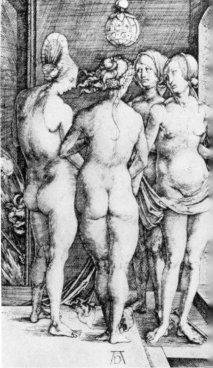

Albert Dürer: The Four Witches.
Source: Montague Summers, *The Geography of Witchcraft,* Routledge and Kegan Paul, London: 1927.

3

Montague Summers'
Compilations

Perhaps the most assiduous student of witchcraft in this century was a learned Jesuit, Montague Summers, the author (among other publications) of the massive *The History of Witchcraft and Demonology* (London, 1926), and *The Geography of Witchcraft* (London, 1927). He also edited English translations (some done by himself) of the works of the demonologists of the sixteenth and seventeenth centuries, published in the nineteen-thirties. It is clear from his comments that he believed that most of these accounts were substantially true. Nonetheless there is plenty of material in what he himself says, let alone in what the old demonologists say, to lend support to a Freudian interpretation of the Witch Craze. Look, for instance, at the following details in his description of the proceedings at the sabbat:

The witches adored Satan, or the Master of the Sabbat who presided in place of Satan, by prostrations, genuflections, gestures, and obeisances. In mockery of solemn bows and seemly courtesies the worshippers of the Demon approach him awkwardly, with grotesque and obscene mops and mows, sometimes straddling sideways, sometimes walking backwards, as Guazzo says: Cum accedunt ad dæmones eos ueneraturi terga obuertunt & cessim eum eanerorum more supplicaturi manus inuersas retro applicant. But their chief act of homage was the reverential kiss, *osculum infame*. This impious and lewd ritual is mentioned in detail by most authorities and is to be found in all lands and centuries. So Delrio writes: 'The Sabbat is presided over by a Demon, the Lord of the Sabbat, who appears in some monstrous form, most generally as a goat or some hound of hell, seated upon a haughty throne. The witches who resort to the Sabbat approach the throne with their backs turned, and worship him . . . and then, as a sign of their homage, they kiss his fundament.' Guazzo notes: 'As a sign of homage witches kiss the Devil's fundament.' And Ludwig Elich says: 'Then as a token of their homage – with reverence be it spoken – they kiss the fundament of the Devil.' 'And at the time when they kiss him under the tail he lets out a wind of very horrible smell,' adds the Spanish *Relacion*, 'fetid, foul, and filthy.'

(*History*, pp. 137–8).

It is not far fetched to presume that such lurid fantasies of celibate theologians were inspired by the desire to degrade and punish women whose mere existence exposed the authors to temptation and the torments of frustrated concupiscence.

The following quotation from Summers' *Geography of Witchcraft* (p. 402) illustrates the frequent connection in the minds of the accusers between witchcraft and sexual ills:

During the reign of Henry IV of France (1589–1610) there are the same lengthy and detailed records, year after year, of witch-trials and executions. In 1597 a certain Chamouillard was hanged and burned for having by his charms rendered a young demoiselle de la Barrière sterile and unable to perform the marriage act: and in the same year Jean Belon, the rector of St Pierre des Lampes, in the diocese of Bourges, was put to death for using evil enchantments. At Riom Vidal de la Porte was condemned as a sorceror by whose spells not only youths, but even dogs, cats, and other animals were rendered impotent.

The link between celibacy and witchcraft is very clear in what Summers tells us about various events in nunneries, of which the following is an example:

The seventeenth century in France is especially remarkable for the number of cases in which convents became the scenes of Witchcraft and demoniac possession. It seemed as though the forces of evil were launching their whole strength against the houses of prayer and contemplation, boldly storming the very citadels of God. As early as 1551 the religious of the convent of Uvertet in the province of Hoorn in Holland were seized with a mysterious malady which was shrewdly suspected to have no natural origin. In a house of Bridgettines near Xante the sisters imagined themselves transformed into various animals and with loud shrieks imitated the bleating of sheep, the squealing of pigs, the lowing of cows, and other strange bestial sounds. The cloisters of Hessimont near Nieumeghe were haunted by a low sweet music which stirred the heart to passionate longings and an agony of sensual desire. About 1560 the nuns of a convent of Nazareth at Cologne were suspected by the episcopal visitor to be obsessed. Upon examination they avowed that the convent was the resort of incubi with whom they indulged in the most unbridled licentiousness. It was, in fact, proved that many of them had been deflowered, but their paramours were never traced. The ecclesiastical authorities, sore grieved and alarmed, treated the guilty with the utmost severity. At Hensberg, in the duchy of Cleves, the sisters complained of having seen men, who glided along the corridors noiselessly and vanished like shadows, in the actual clausura where no man could possibly be.

The director of this convent, at Aix, a priest of an intensely mystical turn of mind, was a converted Huguenot, Father Romillon. During the year 1609 he took note that Sister Madeleine, and another nun, Louise Capel, who seems to have been one of the few inmates not of aristocratic birth, were attacked by a strange disorder, which did not yield to any natural remedies. So hideous were their convulsions, so extravagant their gestures, that the good priest determined to exorcise them, which he accordingly did in the sacristy of the chapel, so that no scandal might be given. The two patients fell into the most terrible paroxysms as the words of the ritual were pronounced; their cries and screams filled the assistants with horror; now they yelled in piercing tones, now howled with a deep gruff clamour that could hardly be believed to issue from the throats of two frail women. Madeleine at length fell into a comatose trance and averred that she was possessed by Beelzebub, Leviathan, Verrine, and many other devils, to whom she had succumbed owing to the incantations of a priest of Marseilles, Louis Gaufridi. She further alleged that he had debauched when she was but a child of nine years, and that she had been compelled by him to nameless infamy and debauch.

Louis Gaufridi was born at Beauvezer, a village of Colmars, situate on the right bank of the river Verdon, in 1572. He was educated by his uncle, Christophe Gaufridi, a priest of Pouvrières, from whose care he passed to Marseilles, where he distinguished himself by his eagerness for study and a memory unusually retentive and adroit. It would seem that these qualities, to which must be added a handsome face and elegant manners, recommended to the notice of M. de Demandols, who possessed estates which were bordered by the Verdon. Soon after his ordination he was appointed vicar of Accoules (Marseilles), and here he had opportunity for constant intercourse with Madeleine de la Palud, who was his penitent, and whom he sacrilegiously violated whilst she was yet a child.

When after some eighteen months Father Romillon found himself unable to free the two nuns, he appealed to the saintly Sebastian Michaelis, a Dominician of great learning and authority, who was then at St Maximin. By his advice the sisters were brought to the sacred grotto, La Sainte-Baume, hallowed by the tears and penances of S. Mary Magdalen, and there exorcised by Father Francis Domptius, O.P., who was reputed to be well skilled in these matters. Again and again the possessed launched the same accusations against Gaufridi; there were the same scenes of hideously unnatural agitation and violence, twisted limbs, staring eyes, blanched faces, champing mouths that dripped with foam and poured forth fetid blasphemies and obscenities beyond all human imagining.

On the 19 February 1611, a commission was issued to one de Séguiran, a councillor, to arrest Louis Gaufridi, accused of rape, seduction, magic, sorcery, blasphemy, and other heinous and abominable offences.

Madeleine de la Palud was interrogated during three days, 21, 22, 23 February, by President Thoron when she made the amplest confession concerning witchcrafts of every kind, especially the Sabbat at which she had frequently assisted. There she had worshipped the Prince of the Synagogue (for so the coven was called), a man, Lucifer's lieutenant, in effect Gaufridi himself. All present renounced the Holy Trinity, their baptism, and the Catholic Faith. A banquet was spread at several tables, some of which were piled with goodly viands and wine; upon others was served the roast flesh of newly slain infants. Lewd dances were performed, and bawdy songs sung. Each day of the week had its own sexual observances, proceeding to the most infamous conjunctions. The black mass in honour of Satan was celebrated, sometimes by Gaufridi, sometimes by some other wretch, the Host being often thrown to a dog, and the Sacred Blood being scattered over the vile crew who shouted: 'Sanguis eius super nos et super filios nostros.' Upon one occasion a dog who had been led in to devour the consecrated Species, stretched out his paws in adoration before God's Body and bowed his head, nor could kicks and blows compel him to stir. Several broke in floods of tears and began to bewail their sins, after which it was decreed that in future the Host should be defiled and trodden under foot, but that no dogs should be admitted.

Gaufridi, who was thrown into prison on the 20 February, made a complete avowal of his iniquities, his sorceries and seductions of religious, . . . he was tortured . . . .

On 30 April, Gaufridi was publicly degraded from all ecclesiastical order by Monsignor Turicella, a Florentine, erstwhile confessor to Maria de' Medici, now Bishop of Marseilles, and delivered over to secular justice. About five o'clock in the afternoon he was burned at the stake before an immense concourse of people.

(*Geography*, pp. 402–11)

4
Henri Boguet

One of the most influential instigators of persecutions was Henri Boguet who, as the chief prosecutor, played a leading role in a number of big hunts in France. His treatise was translated into English under the title *An Examen of Witches*. The quotations are from the 1926 reprint:

Let us now examine by what ills witches afflict mankind particularly. I maintain that they afflict people with all kinds of ills of the stomach and the head and the feet, with cholic, paralysis, apoplexy, leprosy, epilepsy, dropsy, strangury, etc. And this they do easily with the help of Satan, who secretly causes persons to swallow certain poisons and drugs; or perhaps the witches themselves mix them with their food and drink. And according to the composition of the poison it will spread over the whole body or attack only one member; for, says Cardan, there are poisons which do not cause death, but continually attack one of the victims' members. Again, according to Theophrastus, the poison may take two, three, or six months to prepare, and the illness of him who is bewitched will continue for a longer or shorter time according to the time taken to collect the ingredients of the drug. Witches very frequently dry up the milk of nurses, apparently by making them swallow a certain powder which they throw in their broth, unless it is Satan himself who plays this trick. They also cause a man's virile member to disappear and be concealed, and then to reappear at their own pleasure. This is widely practised in Germany.

At times also they prevent carnal copulation between a man and a woman by relaxing the nerves and depriving the member of rigidity; at other times they prevent procreation by turning aside or blocking up the seminal ducts so that the semen does not reach the generative cells. And they hold a married couple thus bound for as long as it pleases them, sowing ten thousand other seeds of discord between them besides. . . . those midwives and wise women who are witches are in the habit of offering to Satan the little children which they deliver, and then of killing them, before they have been baptised, by thrusting a large pin into their brains. There have been those who have confessed to having killed more than forty children in this way.

They do even worse; for they kill them while they are yet in their mothers' wombs. This practice is common to all witches, as we find in Nider, who writes that one named Stadlin in the Diocese of Lausanne confessed that he had killed seven children in their mothers' womb by means of an animal which he had buried under the threshold of the house.

Satan couples with witches sometimes in the form of a black man, sometimes in that of some animal, as a dog or a cat or a ram. With Thievenne Paget and Antoine Tornier he lay in the form of a black man; and when he coupled with Jacquema Paget and Antoine Gandillon he took the shape of a black ram with horns: Françoise Secretain confessed that her demon appeared sometimes as a dog, sometimes as a cat, and sometimes as a fowl when he wished to have carnal intercourse with her. For all these reasons I am convinced that there is real and actual copulation between a witch and a demon; for what is there to prevent the Devil, when he has taken the form of an animal, from coition with a witch? In Toulouse and Paris women have been known to make sexual abuse of a natural dog; and it seems to me quite to the point to refer here to the legends of Pasiphaë and other such women.

It is a matter of far greater doubt whether a living being can be born from the coupling of the Devil with a witch. I remember that, when Antoine Tornier and Antoine Gandillon were asked whether they were not afraid of becoming pregnant by the Devil, one answered that she was too old, and the other that God would not permit it. I have read, too, that Satan has sometimes asked a witch whether she wished to become pregnant by him, and that the witch has said that she did not wish it. It seems then that it is possible for issue to come of this coupling; and also there are many examples of such an occurrence, besides the proof which may be drawn from the Book of Genesis, where it is said that the Sons of God lay with the daughters of men, and that there sprang from them a race of giants, a passage which Josephus understands literally. As for examples, we have the English Merlin, who was said to have been born from the union of a demon with a woman: the Huns and the men of Cyprus are also said to spring from certain witches who had intercourse with the Devil: it is also said that Luther was born from the coupling of the Devil with his mother Marguerite. . . .

The witches, then, being assembled in their Synagogue, first worship Satan, who appears to them now in the shape of a big black man and now as a goat; and to do him the greater homage they offer him candles, which burn with a blue flame; then they kiss him on the shameful parts behind. Some kiss him on the shoulder; and at other times he holds up a black image which he requires the witches to kiss, according to Antide Colas, who said that, on kissing it, they offered a candle or burning torch. Jeanne Platet and Clauda Paget said that the Devil gave them these candles, and that after they had offered them they did not know what became of them.

Following this, they dance; and this they do in a ring back to back. Clauda Jamprost and Françoise Secretain have reported that the lame show more eagerness for these dances than do the others; for they said that the lame urged on the others to leap and dance. Now they dance in this manner back to back so that they may not be recognised; but in these days they make use of a different device for the same purpose, which is to mask themselves, according to the confessions of Clauda Paget, named la Foulet. There are also demons which join in these dances in the shape of goats or rams, as we learn from many witches besides those we have just mentioned; and particularly Antoine Tornier observed that, when she danced, a black ram held her up by the hands with his feet, which were, as she said, very hairy, that is to say, rough and rude.

They are not without pipes at these revels, for there are those whose duty it is to provide the dance music. Most often Satan plays upon the flute, and at other times the witches are content to sing with their voices; but they sing at haphazard and in such confusion that one cannot hear the other. Sometimes, but rarely, they dance in couples and at other times one here and another there, and always in confusion; for their dances are such as those of the fairies, which are truly devils in bodily form who had power no long time since.

After the dancing the witches begin to couple with each other and in this matter the son does not spare his mother, nor the brother his sister, nor the father his daughter; but incest is commonly practised. The Persians also believed that, to be a

competent and complete witch and magician, a person must be
born of a mother by her son.

Of son by mother is a witch conceived,
If the foul Persian creed may be believed.

I may safely leave to the imagination the question whether or
not every other kind of lechery known to the world is practised
at the Sabbat: what is even more remarkable is that Satan
becomes an Incubus for the women and a Succubus for the men.
This is a fact to which George and Antoine Gandillon have
testified and, before them, Antoine Tornier, Jacquema Paget and
several others.

These incests and lecheries bring to my mind the practices of
the Euchites and Gnostics. They used to meet together on Good
Friday evening with certain women, who were their sisters and
aunts and cousins, and had carnal connexion with them. Nine
months later, they again met at the same place and, taking the
children that had been born of these incestuous couplings, they
cut them about all over their bodies and collected their blood in
phials, and afterwards burned the bodies. They then mixed the
blood with ashes and made a sauce, with which they seasoned
their food and drink.

After having abandoned themselves to such foul fleshly
pleasures the witches fall to feasting and banqueting. In their
banquets they have various kinds of meats, which differ according to the locality and the rank of those who are assembled. In
our own district the table was covered with butter, cheese and
flesh; Clauda Jamguillaume, Jacquema Paget and some others
said that there was a great cauldron on the fire from which they
all helped themselves to meat. Their drink is sometimes wine
and sometimes water: Antoine Tornier said that she drank wine
from a wooden cup, but the others mentioned nothing but water.
But there is never any salt; for salt is a symbol of immortality,
and is held in bitter abhorrence by the Devil. Moreover, God
commanded that salt should be mingled with every sacrifice or
oblation which is offered to Him; and therefore it is used in
Baptism, which is a sovereign antidote against the power of the
Devil. It may also be said that, since salt is symbolical of wisdom,
God in His hidden purpose does not allow it to be used at the

Sabbat, so that the witches may know that all that they do is sheer folly.

Having finished the banquet, they render to Satan an account of what they have done since the last assembly; and those are the most welcome who have caused the death of the most persons and cattle, who have cast the most spells of illness, and spoiled the most fruit – in short, those who have done the most mischief and wickedness. Others, who have behaved rather more humanely, are hissed and derided by all, are set apart to one side, and are generally beaten and ill treated by their master; and from this arises the proverb that is common among them – 'Do the worst you can, and the Devil will not know what to demand of you.'

But it is far more difficult to believe that Satan can speak through the shameful parts of a woman, or when the person's mouth is shut, or when the tongue is thrust six inches out of the mouth; or that he can speak when he has no body at all, or one formed only of air. Yet this is known to happen; for we read that she who gave answer in the Delphic Oracle spoke through the lower and shameful parts, as did also a woman in Rhodige, an Italian town mentioned by Cœlius Rhodiginus in his disquisitions.

However, this thing is caused in a natural manner, just as if the voice were formed by an agitation and vibration of air; and it follows that Satan can in this way create a voice, seeing that he is well able to form a body out of air. The echo gives us an example of this, when we see valleys and hollow places reply articulately to the human voice so exactly that it seems as if those places were imitating our speech; and from this it is easy to understand that the human voice may be quite well counterfeited without the use of lungs, tongue or teeth.

It remains for us to show that it is not out of place for our priests to use perfumes in their exorcisms; and this will be very easy. I will readily admit that perfume has no direct virtue against the Evil Spirit, since he has no body and consequently no sense of smell: yet it must be granted me that this wicked Serpent is very glad to find in the bodies of men humours which the more dispose them to be tormented by him, the chief of these being the melancholoy humour, which is of its nature apt to be heavy and sad; and therefore we find that those of a melancholy humour are more often possessed by a devil than are other men.

Now it is certain that there are perfumes which consume and correct these humours, for even sulphur works in a very subtle manner to that effect; and therefore I conclude that the Devil will be more easily cast out of a demoniac's body if it be purged of the humours of which we have just spoken, than if it be still charged with them.

(pp. 28, 32, 55, 69, 89, 92, 189, 190)

5
Nicolas Remy

Nicolas Remy was one of the biggest butchers and torturers but he presents himself (and perhaps saw himself) as a defender of people threatened by witches: engaged in what in modern parlance would be described as a combination of police duties with preventive medicine. The extracts are taken from the old English translation of his *Demonolatry*, reprinted in 1930 by John Rodker, London.

The way to injury and loss is always easy, whereas the road to well-being and safety is beset with every kind of difficulty and obstacle. Similarly, when witches desire to cause sickness or death everything is ready to their hand; for they have the opportunity, every sort of poison, curse, charms and spells, and the Demon himself, the deviser and author of all evil, who never fails them when they summon him; but when it is a question of healing a sickness or saving a life, then there is always something to hinder them. For instance, help has already been sought from the priest or the physician or some other source; the sickness was not caused by the witch in question, but by another; as soon as they are put in prison they are entirely deprived of the healing power which they had before from the Demon; they are only permitted to heal on condition that they exchange that benefit for an even greater loss or injury; they have not been clearly asked in so many words to effect a cure. Such are among the excuses which they always offer for their delays and subterfuges in the matter of healing. The following examples will make this clearer.

Roses Girardine, at Essey, Nov. 1586, asserted for a fact that no disease could be cured except by the witch who had caused it; for none of them was allowed to thrust her sickle into another's corn. Thus the evil is to be feared, and the remedy to be sought, both from the same source. Dominique Euraea, at Charmes, Nov. 1584, said that it was impossible to restore a sick man to health unless his sickness was transferred in an aggravated form to another, and that such an exchange was always the source of some greater evil.

Catharina Gillotia, Huecourt, May 1591, was asked what was the reason that Canassia Godefreda had not recovered from the disease which she had brought upon her by witchcraft, although she had often given her apples and plums and other things to eat which she had successfully used in curing others; and she answered that it was because Godefreda had not first begged her to heal her. Balial Basolus, of Saint Nicolas des Preys de Verdun, March 1587, and Colette Fischer, of Gerbeville, March 1588, mentioned a new kind of obstacle; saying that if a man afflicted in this way were to make and perform a vow to any of the Saints without having told or consulted with them, this contempt of them prevented them from doing anything further to heal the sickness. But it must be suspected that this obstacle is a fiction engendered by their desire for gain or thanks, for which they are above all things eager. For witches make it their chief business to be asked to perform cures so that they may reap some profit, or at least gratitude; since they are for the most part beggars, who support life on the alms they receive.

The foregoing and the following passages suggest that some of the victims (perhaps many, if not most) were healers (medicine women or men) who were punished for their lack of success, which would be particularly conspicuous during an epidemic.

Now the obstacles which are thus said to prevent a witch from curing the sickness which she has caused are not altogether illogical or unreasonable. For in the first place it is not without design that the Demon pretends that, in effecting a cure, he must have the help of her through whose agency he has previously caused the disease. No one doubts that he could do this alone and single-handed; but he acts as he does so that his well-doing may be diminished and depreciated by placing the power of performing it at the pleasure of another; and also that he may earn a greater reputation with his disciples for his service to them, when he shows that he will not without consulting them alter anything of which they have been the authors; for it is no small source of gratification to a witch to know that she is accredited with powers of life and death over mankind; and that when she has cast an evil spell upon a man, it will not be

removed by any other means than, or before the time that, she
herself shall have determined upon.

Secondly, as to their allegation that they cannot effect a cure
except upon an untouched subject who has not already sought
physical relief from a physician or spiritual salvation from a
priest; here also there is some fraudulent and malicious fiction,
since in neither of those cases is the Demon likely to earn any
reward for his cure. Therefore this obstacle proceeds rather from
the Demon's jealousy and his fear that he would get no credit
for a cure which would probably be attributed to another agent
who had preceded him. Therefore they take the greatest pains
to inculcate in those whom they have bewitched with a sickness
the belief that they must shun all remedies, human and divine,
if they wish to recover, and that if they even think of having
recourse to such remedies they must certainly lose all hope of
ever regaining their health. There is always this further motive,
that the Demon wishes to avoid indulging the pity of his
disciples, if indeed they are ever moved by pity.

And thirdly, as to their being hindered by the fact of their
accusation and imprisonment, I would not deny that this is true
in the case of those who by confessing their sins and by penitence
have driven the Demon from them; for then the pact is broken
by the terms of which they had received that supernatural power
of healing, and therefore those powers must dwindle and vanish.
There can be no more convincing proof of this than the fact that
those in that condition have no more power to cast injurious
spells, however much they may wish to, not even upon the very
torturers who put them to the question. Moreover, it has often
been proved that when the Judge, from a wish to put this matter
to the test, by a mere nod or a word discharges them, they have
at once flown away and, re-entering the Demon's household as
it were by right of postliminy, have performed many stupendous
prodigies. But if with contumacious obstinacy they persist in
denying their guilt; or if they do not in so many words and after
the customary form forswear the society of the Demon and
renege his friendship, or rather abjure their fealty to him and
shake off his yoke: in that case I should say that their allegation
is false, that they are no longer able to do anything under his
auspices, particularly if it is a matter of restoring a man to health.
For even when they are in chains in their prison cells their
Demons often visit them, awake in them a hope of freedom,

give them their advice and offer them their services; and are in every respect as favourable, indulgent and helpful to them as they ever were before: so that it is not likely that they would refuse to heal a sickness for them if they asked them, and if it were safe for them to make such a request. Moreover, it is foolish to say that the witch is prevented by his chains, while the Demon, who has no need of the witch's co-operation, is in no way bound or in chains. And there is no Judge who would think of putting any obstacle or hindrance in the way of so salutary a deed, if it lay at all within his discretion.

Nicole Morèle's father, at Serre, Jan. 1587, was charged with witchcraft and was pleading his cause in prison, and something that he said brought his daughter also under suspicion of that crime. Consequently, the Apparitor, who was then present, persuaded the Judge to have her arrested. Her Demon informed Morèle of this while she was still at liberty, and urged her to take some vengeance on the Apparitor for that injury, saying that he would gladly undertake the execution of it if she asked him. She agreed, and he at once flew to the Apparitor's house, where he found his wife sitting by the fire giving her baby the breast, and passing by her he dusted her breasts with so venomous a powder that they were immediately dried up and lost all their milk. The Apparitor easily suspected the cause of this and went to Morèle, who was now in prison, and giving her a nicely cooked millet cake to appease her, asked her not to refuse him any help that she could give in this matter; for in return he would take care that she lacked for nothing to make her life easy while she was in prison: after which he went out, waiting to see what she would do. The Demon immediately appeared and chid her bitterly for having had converse with the Apparitor; but at last he allowed himself to be persuaded to restore the milk to his wife, even to superfluity if she so desired; and this he soon afterwards did by secretly dusting her with a white powder.

Catharine Ocray at Nancy, 1584, had been released on her own bail, but was again thrown into prison both on account of fresh suspicions against her, and by the strictest command of our Most Serene Prince, in an audience with whom I had unreservedly laid bare the whole facts of this case. When one of the witnesses against her deposed that, before she had been brought back to prison, she had cast a spell upon his arm and withered it, she seized his arm violently as if in anger and, to the great astonishment of all who were present, it was immediately made sound again; and after having been for many months powerless and useless, it became in a moment vigorous and capable of performing all its usual functions as before. This led to a strong suspicion that she maintained her association with her Little Master to the very last; for though she had often been urged to abjure him she had refused to do so, saying that it was impossible to reject one whom you had never admitted. There have been other witches who, though in prison, have prescribed the use of herbs and lotions and unguents and other such remedies, saying that their application to the sick would not be without result.

Lastly, the benefit of such cures is qualified either by some lasting trace of the sickness, or often by its transference with even greater pain and torment to another. This is but another illustration of the fact which we have already so often pointed out, that the Demon never allows his prey to be snatched wholly from his hands, but that there must always be something as the price and reward of his work. Thus when he enters into a pact to serve and work for a man (on which account he is commonly called the man's familiar spirit), he takes care that the chief condition of the pact shall be that within a stated time he shall be free to find a new master, or else to do what he will with his present master.

The Herbs, Powder, Straws, and other such Trash which Witches strew on the Ground are a certain Cause of Death or Illness to those who Walk upon them, provided that it is the Witch's intention and wish to injure them; but those against whom no Evil is contemplated can Walk safe and unharmed over them. And this clearly shows the Cunning and Wile of the Devil in Afflicting and Destroying Men.

It has been shown from the definite assertions of witches that they often use the same instruments for procuring both sickness and healing: that the powder with which they dust the clothes of others is sometimes fatal to them, although the witches themselves may touch it with their hands with impunity; and that the sickness so caused is amenable to almost no cure except such as the witch is willing to provide; and that this cure usually consists in the utterance of one or two words, or a mere hand touch, and often in the application of things which ordinarily have no healing power at all. From all this it is sufficiently clear that there is in the things so used by them no inherent or natural power either of hurting or of healing; but that, whatever prodigious results are effected, it is all done by the Demons through some power of which the source and explanation are not known. For in the examples of such doings we find much that can spring from no probable cause in nature; but that certain substances behave in a manner entirely opposed to that which would normally be expected from their active and passive properties. This will be proved and clearly shown by the following instances.

Odilla Boncourt at Haraucourt, Dec. 1586, said that it was the practice of witches, when they are afraid of being detected in their crime, to scatter a poison powder on the path which they thought would be taken by those whose misfortune they were plotting. And this is borne out by the confession of Rosa Gerardine at Essey, Nov. 1586, that she had brought a fatal sickness upon her comrade Stephanus Obertus by scattering such a powder on his threshold before dawn. Jacobus Agathius at Laach, March 1588, said that the Demon had suggested the same means to him as by far the easiest way to rid himself of the wife of Hilary le Ban. Isabella Bardaea at Epinal, May 1588, and Martha Mergelatia said that they had never failed in such an attempt against anyone; especially if they had acted at the instigation of their Demon.

For just as of all living creatures their lust is chiefly to kill men, so of human creatures witches take an especial delight in the slaughter of infants and those who by virtue of their age are innocent and guiltless. This fact is exemplified in the behaviour of Jacoba Cavallia, that Drigie mentioned above, and Odilla, who, as I remember, had an excessive tax (according to their own computation) imposed upon them by the assessors of the village in which they lived, and wished to be avenged for that injustice by some signal act of retribution. The Demon did not fail to provide them with an apt and convenient means of attaining their wish by scattering their poison as thickly as possible on the grazing grounds of the cattle of that village; and, to remove their last difficulty, he told them that they could easily prepare the necessary poison by pounding up the first worms that they found until they were reduced to a powder fine enough to sprinkle. When, therefore, they had acted accordingly, within a few days there perished in that village a hundred and fifty head of cattle, as Drigie said, or a hundred and sixty according to Odilla's account; for they were questioned separately, and agreed in everything except the numbers. The truth of their statements was attested by the facts themselves; for at about the time indicated that number of cattle was lost by the villagers.

Notice that the herbs, dust, worms and other such trash scattered about by witches do not only cause sickness or death, against which defensive measures can be taken when they are conveyed by contagion as in the case of the breathing or touching of plague-infested matters; but they also break or weaken limbs, and diminish, draw off and dry up the milk in the breasts. It is obvious that such effects can only proceed from some secret co-operation of the Demon. This conviction is strengthened by the fact that these matters are harmful only to those against whom they are intentionally directed; whilst everyone else can walk over them and tread upon them safely and without experiencing any hurt. This is proved beyond doubt by the following perform-ance of Alexée Drigie (Haraucourt, Nov. 1586).

Her Demon gave her a handful of fern to scatter on the path most frequently used by the daughter of a shepherd named Claude, of whom she was jealous, so that she might suddenly die. But her one fear was lest this calamity should befall others also who went that way, whom she had no wish to injure. The Demon, however, told her to be at ease on that score, since the poison would affect no one except her for whom it was intended; and it happened just as he had said. For of all those who passed by that way, only that shepherd's daughter met her death because of it. Not long afterwards the same witch miserably afflicted the health of Humbert the Castellan by rubbing his couch with the same powder; but the charm was deadly to him alone; for many others, both before and after him, had sat on that couch.

Away with them, then, away with all who say that the talk of a pact between witches and Demons is mere nonsense; for the facts themselves give them the lie, and are attested and proved by the legitimate complaints of many men. But some are so obstinate as to be unable to preceive this; they are such double fools that no misfortune can bring them wisdom.

It is a fact that all witches who make a Demon free of their bodies (and this they all do when they enter his service, and it is as it were the first pledge of their pact with him) are completely in agreement in saying that, if the Demon emits any semen, it is so cold that they recoil with horror on receiving it. In Psellus, *De Daemonibus*, Marcus makes the same statement: 'If they ejaculate any semen it is, like the body from which it comes, so lacking in warmth that nothing can be more unfit or unsuitable for procreation.'

I need not here run through all the arguments which are usually adduced in support of this opinion; for the fact is proved by actual experience. Alexander ab Alexandro (*Genialium dierum*, II, 9) records that he knew a man who told him that the appearance of a friend who had lately died (but it is probable that this was a spectral illusion of a Demon) came to him, very pale and wasted, and tried to get into bed with him: and although he fought with him and prevented him from doing this, he yet succeeded in inserting one foot, which was so cold and rigid that no ice could be compared with it. Cardan also tells a similar story of a friend of his who went to bed in a chamber which had formerly been notoriously haunted by Demons, and felt the touch of an icily cold hand. But to come nearer home, the confession of Ponsète of Essey, who was convicted of witchcraft at Montlhéry (4th April, 1583), agrees with what has been said above. She said that whenever, as is the way of lovers, she put her hand in her Demon's bosom she felt it as hard and rigid as marble.

Averroës, Blessed Albertus Magnus, and several others add to the above two methods of procuring this monstrous procreation a third which is perhaps more credible and probable. According to them, the Demons inject as Incubi the semen which they have previously received as Succubi; and this view can reasonably be supported by the fact that this method differs from the natural and customary way of men only in respect of a very brief intermission in its accomplishment. This objection, moreover, they easily overcome by quoting the extraordinary skill of Demons in preserving matters from their natural dissolution. But whether it be a man or a woman who is concerned, in either case the work of nature must be free, and there must be nothing to delay or impede it in the very least. If shame, fear, horror or some stronger feeling is present, all that comes from the loins is spent in vain and nature becomes sterile; and for this reason the very consummation of love and carnal warmth which it implies will act as a spur to the accomplishment of the venereal act. But all they who have spoken to us of their copulations with Demons agree in saying that nothing colder or more unpleasant could be imagined or described. At Dalheim, Pétrone of Armentières declared that, as soon as he embraced his *Abrahel*, all his limbs at once grew stiff. Hennezel at Vergaville, July 1586, said that it was as if he had entered an ice-bound cavity, and that he left his *Schwartzburg* with the matter unaccomplished. (These were the names of their Succubas.) And all female witches maintain that the so-called genital organs of their Demons are so huge and so excessively rigid that they cannot be admitted without the greatest pain. Alexée Drigie (at Haraucourt, 10th Nov., 1586) reported that her Demon's penis, even when only half in erection, was as long as some kitchen utensils which she pointed to as she spoke; and that there were neither testicles nor scrotum attached to it. Claude Fellet (at Mazières, 2nd Nov., 1584) said that she had often felt it like a spindle swollen to an immense size so that it could not be contained by even the most capacious woman without great pain. This agrees with the complaint of Nicole Morèle (at Serre, 19th Jan., 1587) that, after such miserable copulation, she always had to go straight to bed as if she had been tired out by some long and violent agitation. Didatia of Miremont (at Preny, 31st July, 1588) also said that, although she had many years' experience of men, she was always so stretched by the huge, swollen member of her Demon that the sheets were drenched with blood. And nearly all witches protest that it is wholly against their will that they are embraced by Demons, but that it is useless for them to resist.

Therefore I think that it is manifest and plain enough that such copulation cannot so titillate the nerves as to evoke any semen; and everyone knows that without semen there can be no procreation. But let us assume that there are those whose lust can be aroused by such frigid and joyless embraces, and that the Demon can find here a man and there a woman of such sort; and let us grant that he goes from one to the other with great speed like a stage tumbler: even though the delay involved is of the shortest, the vital element must surely be lacking for the accomplishment of so great a matter as propagation. Physicians say that no coupling can have fertile results unless the male member penetrates to the necessary place, for the seed must be discharged in one place and must not be spent or dissipated on the way. For we suppose that as Plutarch records in his *Moralia* Zeno was right in saying that semen is a mixture extracted from all the forces of life, and that it loses all its potency and virtue unless it has a straight and uninterrupted passage to the womb. Therefore Galen (*De usu partium*, XV) said that a man's yard must be at its most rigid in the act of coition so that the semen may be carried as far as possible. For even though the semen may be fertile it is entirely incapable of procreation if it cannot be deeply enough injected, as happens in the case of those who are too quickly brought to the crisis.

Demons do not perform this act for the purpose of raising issue, or in order to give or receive any pleasure . . . Their purpose is rather, by the practice of such lewdness, to sink deeper and deeper into iniquity those whom they have once ensnared.

Granted the above premises and postulates, it is not, I think, absurd to say that the birth of such monstrous and deformed children is due to the fact that, at the conception or during the formation of the child, its mother has had frequent intercourse with a Demon, the sight of whom has so strongly worked upon her imagination as to affect the appearance of the child. As for their savage utterance and their unnatural gait and running about, these are altogether from the Demon who, independently of the mother's will, has entered into the living child in the womb or into such as are untimely born through abortion. And this, as Alexander ab Alexandro says (*Genialium dierum*, II, 25, and V, 27), is the reason why such infants were formerly thrown into a river or the sea, or else banished to the ends of the earth. And at the present time the Church considers them unfit to receive Christian baptism, and we take care to smother them to death as soon as they are born; doubtless because they carry suspicion of the hidden presence of a Demon lurking within them.

It is, then, most certain that such are the issue of men, not of Demons, even though their shape and entire composition may seem hardly human. Cicero says (*De finibus bon. & mal.*, I) that to understand the nature of anything, two points are to be considered: first, the material from which a thing is made; second, the force by which it is made. Now both of these are in the control of man, whereas neither of them is at the effective command of a Demon in the matter of such procreation. It is useless for certain men of ill-employed leisure to maintain to us that such geminate and hybrid births are due to external and adventitious causes. In short, to return to the point from which we digressed, there seems more truth in the opinion of those who deny that such procreation is due to the borrowing (if I may call it) of semen by Demons. Yet I know that the contrary opinion is held by many learned authors with whom it would seem rash to disagree if this were a question of religion or sacred matters; but since it does not touch the principles of faith, and even the Fathers treat the matter as purely problematical, I do not think that I have at all placed my orthodoxy in question by a free exposition of the reasons which have led me to favour one opinion rather than any other.

(pp. 9, 12, 13, 15, 16, 19, 58, 59, 60, 117, 118, 119, 120)

6

Francesco Guazzo

Unlike Remy, Francesco Maria Guazzo was a theoretician rather than practitioner of the persecution. His treatise was published in 1593. As the reader can see, Guazzo (like the other writers) was fully acquainted with natural explanations of disease.

The extracts are taken from the 1929 reprint of *Compendium Maleficarum* by John Rodker, translated by E. A. Ashwin.

Avicenna and Galen and Hippocrates deny that it is possible for any diseases to be brought upon man by demons; and their view is followed by Pietro Pomponazzi and Levin Lemne not because they did not believe that the demons, which they acknowledged to be evil, wished to cause disease, but because they held that every disease is due to natural causes. But that is no good argument: for is it not possible for sickness to spring from natural causes, and at the same time possible for demons to be the instigators of such sicknesses?

Did not the devil afflict Job with loathsome sores from the soles of his feet to the crown of his head? Did not the devil put to an alien use the tongue and ears of him whom S. Matthew calls the Lunatic? Did not a devil afflict Saul with a black humour? The account is quite explicit, for it says that an evil spirit afflicted him, which went away when David played the harp.

Let us now see by what method the demon causes sickness. This has been clearly set forth by Franciscus Valesius, who says that the demon is the external cause of sickness when he comes from without to inhabit a body and bring diseases to it; and if the sickness has some material source he sets in motion its inner causes. Thus he induces the melancholy sickness by first disturbing the black bile in the body and so dispersing a black humour throughout the brain and the inner cells of the body: and this black bile he increases by superinducing other irritations and by preventing the purging of the humour. He brings epilepsy, paralysis and such maladies by a stoppage of the heavier physical fluids, obstructing and blocking the ventricle of the brain and the nerve-roots. He causes blindness or deafness, bringing a noxious secretion in the eyes or ears. Often again he suggests ideas to the imagination which induce love or hatred or other mental disturbances. For the purpose of causing bodily infirmities he distils a spirituous substance from the blood itself, purifies it of all base matter, and uses it as the aptest, most efficacious and swiftest weapon against human life: I say that from the most potent poisons he extracts a quintessence with which he infects the very spirit of life, and . . . so establishes his devil-made disease that human skill is hardly able to find a remedy, since the devil's poison is too subtle and tenuous, too swift and sure in killing, and reaches to the very marrow of the bones. But those more common maladies which are caused solely by some external injury or noxious breath, by means of certain instruments of witchcraft, unguents, signs, buried charms and such things, have no natural power for evil in themselves, but are merely symbols in response to which the demon fulfils his pact with a witch.

A certain honest woman who had been legally married to one of the household of the Archduke formally deposed the following in the presence of a Notary. In the time of her maidenhood she had been in the service of one of the citizens, whose wife became afflicted with grievous pains in the head; and a woman came who said she could cure her, and so began certain incantations and rites. And I carefully watched (said this woman) what she did, and saw that, against the nature of water poured into a vase, she caused water to rise in its vessel together with other ceremonies which there is no need to mention. And considering that the pains in my mistress's head were not assuaged by these means, I addressed the witch in some indignation with these words: 'I do not know what you are doing, but whatever it is, it is witchcraft, and you are doing it for your own profit.' Then the witch at once replied: 'You will know in three days whether I am a witch or not.' And so it proved; for on the third day when I sat down and took up a spindle, I suddenly felt a terrible pain in my body. First it was inside me, so that it seemed that there was no part of my body in which I did not feel horrible shooting pains; then it seemed to me just as if burning coals were being continually heaped upon my head; thirdly, from the crown of my head to the soles of my feet there was no place large enough for a pinprick that was not covered with a rash of white pustules;

and so I remained in these pains, crying out and wishing only for death, until the fourth day. At last my mistress's husband told me to go to a certain tavern; and with great difficulty I went, whilst he walked before, until we were in front of the tavern. 'See!' he said to me; 'there is a loaf of white bread over the tavern door.' 'I see,' said I. Then he said: 'Take it down, if you possibly can; for it may do you good.' And I, holding on to the door with one hand as much as I could, got hold of the loaf with the other. 'Open it' (said my master) 'and look carefully at what is inside.' Then, when I had broken open the loaf, I found many things inside it, especially some white grains very like the pustules on my body; and I saw also some seeds and herbs such as I could not eat or even look at, with the bones of serpents and other animals. In my astonishment I asked my master what was to be done; and he told me to throw it all into the fire. I did so; and behold! suddenly, not in an hour or even a few minutes, but at the moment when that matter was thrown into the fire, I regained all my former health.

The same author tells in the same place the following story. An honest married woman deposed the following on oath. Behind my house (she said) I have a greenhouse, and my neighbour's garden borders on it. One day I noticed that a passage had been made from my neighbour's garden to my greenhouse, not without some damage being caused; and as I was standing in the door of my greenhouse reckoning to myself and bemoaning both the passage and the damage, my neighbour suddenly came up and asked if I suspected her. But I was frightened because of her bad reputation, and only answered, 'The footprints on the grass are a proof of the damage.' Then she was indignant because I had not, as she hoped, accused her with actionable words, and went away murmuring; and though I could hear her words, I could not understand them. After a few days I became very ill with pains in the stomach, and the sharpest twinges shooting from my left side to my right, and conversely, as if two swords or knives were thrust through my breast; whence day and night I disturbed all the neighbours with my cries. And when they came from all sides to console me, it happened that a certain clay-worker, who was engaged in an adulterous intrigue with that witch, my neighbour, coming to visit me, took pity on my illness, and after a few words of comfort went away. But the next day he returned in a hurry, and, after consoling me, added: 'I am going to test whether your illness is due to witchcraft, and if I find that it is, I shall restore your health.' So he took some molten lead and, while I was lying in bed, poured it into a bowl of water which he placed on my body. And when the lead solidified into a certain image and various shapes, he said: 'See! your illness has been caused by witchcraft; and one of the instruments of that witchcraft is hidden under the threshold of your house door. Let us go, then, and remove it, and you will feel better." So my husband and he went to remove the charm; and the clay-worker, taking up the threshold, told my husband to put his hand into the hole which then appeared, and take out whatever he found; and he did so. And first he brought out a waxen image about a palm long, perforated all over, and pierced through the sides with two needles, just in the same way that I felt the stabbing pains from side to side; and then little bags containing all sorts of things, such as grains and seeds and bones. And when all these things were burned, I became better, but not entirely well. For although the shootings and twinges stopped, and I quite regained my appetite for food, yet even now I am by no means fully restored to health. And when we asked her why it was that she had not been completely restored, she answered: There are some other instruments of witchcraft hidden away which I cannot find. And when I asked the man how he knew where the first instruments were hidden, he answered: 'I knew this through the love which prompts a friend to tell things to a friend.'

How to Distinguish Demoniacs, and Those who are Simply Bewitched

The peculiar symptoms of possession by demons through witchcraft are difficult to recognise when the demon which has been sent into a person by witchcraft mingles himself with some unclean substance introduced into the body from another source, or arising from the humours of the sick person himself. For as long as such substance remains hidden in any part of the body, it often happens that there are no signs of its presence beyond some interference with the natural functions of that particular part. Many such persons however, have debased imaginations, especially in their sleep, and so betray the presence of a demon: but this indication by itself is not enough, since it is common also to sufferers from melancholia. But when the evil spirit moves from one place to another in the body, the matter becomes easier to recognise; as follows:

1. If something moves about the body like a live thing, so that the possessed feel as it were ants crawling under their skin.

2. If the part of the body for which the demon is making is stirred by a sort of palpitation.

3. If the patient is tortured with certain prickings.

4. If it is as though wind descended from his head to his feet, and then again went from his feet to his head.

5. If blisters are raised upon the tongue and immediately disappear; or if they are like many little grains, it is a sign that he is inhabited by many demons.

6. If the demon rises as far as the throat and causes it to swell, and brings on a dry cough.

7. If the demon takes hold of his tongue and twists it and makes it swell; or if he causes it to give utterance not to the man's thoughts but to those of the demon; or if the mouth is stretched wide open and the tongue thrust out.

8. If he feels as if cold water were continually being poured down his back.

9. An even more certain sign is when the sick man speaks in foreign tongues unknown to him, or understands others speaking in those tongues; or when, being but ignorant, the patients argue about high and difficult questions; or when they discover hidden and long-forgotten matters, or future events, or the secrets of the inner conscience, such as the sins and imaginings of the bystanders; or if they provoke them to quarrel without cause or become so furious that they cannot be bound or restrained by many strong men.

10. Some say that they hear a voice speaking inside them, but that they know nothing of the meaning of the words.

11. Others, when they are asked what they have done or said, confess that they remember nothing afterwards.

12. Some think that it is an infallible and inseparable sign when those who are possessed are unable to attend Divine worship, so that they can by no means be sprinkled with Holy Water, nor hear nor utter sacred words: but if they are compelled by force to observe the ceremonies of the Church or the Divine Offices, and chiefly if they are forced to be present at the most Holy Sacrifice of the Altar, then they are tormented far more violently. And in support of this opinion is the fact that they

themselves testify that they wish to assist and be present at all these Masses and Offices, and to have the help of holy things, but that there is something within them which strongly prevents them.

13. Some demoniacs have terrible eyes; and the demons miserably destroy their limbs and kill their bodies unless help is quickly brought to them.

14. Some pretend to be stupid, and always grow even more so; but they can be detected if they refuse to recite the Psalm *Miserere mei Deus*, or *Qui habitat in adiutorio Altissimi*, or the beginning of the Gospel of S. John, *In principio erat Uerbum*, or similar passages of Scripture.

15. It is a sign of obsession if a man speak in a tongue foreign to his own country, provided that he is not living out of his own country.

16. It is a manifest sign when an ignorant man speaks literary and grammatical Latin, or if without knowledge of the art he sings musically or says something of which he could never have had any knowledge.

17. Abstinence from food and drink for seven or more days is a powerful sign.

18. When some inner power seems to urge the possessed to hurl himself from a precipice, or hang or strangle himself, or the like.

19. Sometimes they become as if they were stupid, blind, lame, deaf, dumb, lunatic, and almost incapable of movement, whereas before they were active, could speak, hear and see, and in other respects acted sensibly.

20. It is also a sign when they are subject to sudden frights, which are as suddenly allayed.

21. A man may very surely be known for a demoniac if he is disturbed when the exorcisms are read.

22. When the priest's hand is placed upon his head, it feels very heavy and ponderous.

23. When the patient feels under the priest's hand something as cold as ice.

24. When a very cold wind descends through his shoulders and reins.

25. When his head swells to an enormous size.

26. When his brain feels as if it were tightly bound, or pierced and stricken as if by a sword.

27. When the head and face, and sometimes the whole body, swells as if it were filled with hot vapour.

28. Some are afflicted with violent fever and headache, and their whole body is weakened and in pain; but all these symptoms last a very little while, since a conjuration takes away the power of the demon.

29. In some the throat is so constricted that they seem as if they are being strangled.

30. From the abdominal orifice of some there issue certain matters like balls, as if they were worms or ants or frogs.

31. Some have a great vomiting from their stomachs.

32. Many feel acute pain in their guts.

33. The stomach of some becomes forcibly inflated.

34. Some feel a contraction of the heart, as if it had been unmercifully beaten.

35. Sometimes the demon shows himself in some part of the body palpitating like a fish, or like moving ants.

36. Sometimes the bewitched person has a face the colour of cedar wood.

37. Some have very narrow eyes, and appear bound in all their limbs, and their shoulder blades grate dryly.

38. Two very sure signs are the contraction of the heart and of the arms, and when it seems to them that they have a lump upon their stomach.

39. Some have their hearts punctured as if by needles.

40. Some feel as if their heart was being eaten away.

41. Some have great pain in their heart and kidneys, and it seems as if those organs were being torn by dogs.

42. Some feel a lump rising and falling in their throat.

43. In some the genital vein is obstructed.

44. Some are so indisposed in their stomachs that they vomit whatever they eat and drink; but this is a very slight sign unless accompanied by other symptoms.

45. Some have a very cold wind, or one as hot as fire running through their stomach.

46. In some the sign is indigestion of their food; especially when they are given drugs without being relieved.

47. Some have a continuous pulsation about their necks, which seems to inspire them with terror.

The Signs which Show a Man to be Simply Bewitched

All the above have been far more exactly classified and proved by Codronchi (*De morbis ueneficis*, III, 13) who states that some of those signs are common to all cases of bewitchment, and others peculiar to particular cases. He says that the signs common to all cases are to be found either in the cause of the malady or in its concomitant circumstances. Such signs may be recognised in the cause, when the sickness originates from some inordinate and irrational love or some insensate hatred for another, or from the curses or threats of some witch, or if magic charms are found such as we have often spoken of and are mentioned by Andrea Cesalpini (*De inuestigat, daemonum*. c. 22). Among the signs which accompany the sickness are paroxysms, and the efficacy or harmfulness of medicines. The commonest signs are the following:

1. In the first place, when the patient's sickness is very difficult to diagnose, so that the physicians hesitate and are in doubt and keep changing their minds, and are afraid to make any definite pronouncement about it.

2. If, although remedies have been applied from the very first, the sickness does not abate but rather increases and grows worse.

3. If it does not, like natural sicknesses, come on by degrees; but the sick man often suffers the severest symptoms and pains from the very beginning, although there is no apparent pathological cause for it.

4. That the sickness is very erratic: and although it may be periodic, it does not keep its regular periods; and although it may resemble a natural sickness, yet it differs in many respects.

5. Although the sick man is often in the greatest pain, he cannot say in which part he feels the pain.

6. At times the sick give the most mournful sighs without any manifest cause.

7. Some lose their appetite, and some vomit up their food and are so sick in the stomach that often they are doubled up with pain, and a sort of lump may be seen rising and falling from the stomach to the throat; and if they try to eject this when it is risen all their efforts are in vain, although it may very soon shoot out of its own accord.

8. They feel painful pricks in the region of the heart, so that often they say that it is being torn in two.

9. In some the pulse may be seen beating and, as it were, trembling in their necks.

10. Others have excruciating pains in their neck or kidneys or the bottom of their bellies, and often an ice-cold wind goes about their stomach and quickly comes again, or they feel a vapour like a hot flame of fire tormenting them in the same manner.

11. Some become sexually impotent.

12. Some fall into a light sweat especially at night, although the weather and the season are very cold.

13. Others seem to have certain parts of their bodies twisted as it were in a knot.

14. The sicknesses with which those who are bewitched suffer are generally a wasting or emaciation of the whole body and a loss of strength, together with a deep languor, dullness of mind, various melancholy ravings, different kinds of fever, all of which keep the physicians very busy; certain convulsive movements of an epileptic appearance; a sort of rigidity of the limbs giving the appearance of a fit: sometimes the head swells in all directions, or such a weakness pervades the whole body that they can hardly move on any account at all.

15. Sometimes the whole skin, but generally only the face, becomes yellow or ashen coloured.

16. Some have their eyelids so tight shut that they can scarcely open them, and there are certain tests by which such may be recognised.

17. Those who are bewitched can hardly bear to look at the face of a priest, at least not directly; for they keep shifting the whites of the eyes in different ways.

18. When the charms are burned, the sick are wont to change for the worse, or to take some greater or less harm according as their bewitchment was slight or severe; so that not infrequently they are forced to utter terrible cries and roars. But if no change or fresh lesion can be found, there will be great hope that the sick man will with a little attention be presently restored to good health.

19. If by chance the witch should come to see the sick man, the patient is at once affected with great uneasiness and seized with terror and trembling. If it is a child, it' cries. The eyes become grey in colour, and other remarkable changes are to be noted in the sick man.

20. Finally when the priest, to heal the sickness, applies

certain holy liniments to the eyes, ears, brow, and other parts, if a sweat or some other change is seen in those parts it is a sign that he is bewitched.

The following is the usual practice to determine whether the sick man is possessed by a demon. They secretly apply to the sick man a writing with the sacred words of God, or Relics of the Saints, or a blessed Agnus Dei, or some other holy thing. The priest places his hand and his stole upon the head of the possessed and pronounces sacred words. Thereupon the sick man begins to shake and tremble, and in his pain makes many uncouth movements, and says and does many strange things. If the demon is in his head, he feels the keenest pains in his head, or else his head and his face are suffused with a hot red glow like fire. If he is in his eyes, he twists them about. If in the back, he bruises his limbs before and behind, and sometimes makes the whole body so rigid and inflexible that no exertion of force can bend it.

Sometimes they fall down as if dead, as though they were suffering from tertiary epilepsy, and a sort of vapour rushes up into their heads: but at the priest's bidding they arise, and the vapour returns whence it came. If the demon is in their throats, they are so throttled as to be nearly strangled. If he is in the nobler parts of the body, as about the heart or lungs, he causes panting, palpitation and syncope. If he is more towards the stomach, he provokes hiccoughs and vomiting so that sometimes they cannot take food, or if they do they cannot retain it. And he causes them to void a sort of ball by the back passage, with roarings and other harsh cries; and afflicts them with the wind and pain about the midriff. They are known also sometimes by certain fumes of sulphur or some other strong smelling matter.

I find that learned men have given seven immediate causes of impotence. The first is when one of a married couple is made hateful to the other, or both hateful to each other, by means of calumny or suspicion, or by the affliction of some disease, as Medea is said to have injected a poison which made all the women of Lemnos smell badly in their breath, and so caused their husbands to neglect them.

The second is some bodily hindrance to their coming together. By this means a husband and wife are either kept apart in different places; or, when they try to approach each other, a phantasm or some such thing is interposed between them, as will be seen in the example.

The third is when the vital spirit is hindered from flowing to the genital organ, and so the emission of semen is prevented. This has been well expounded by John Mayor.

The fourth is when the fertile semen is dried up and taken away.

The fifth is when the man's penis becomes flabby whenever he wishes to perform the conjugal act.

The sixth is the application of certain drugs which in some way deprive a woman of the power to conceive. These are the more common causes mentioned by learned Doctors.

The seventh is rarer, namely, the closing up or narrowing of the female genitals; or the retraction, hiding or actual removal of the male genitals. Sprenger (II, q. i, cap. 7) and Remy (II, 5) tell various stories of such a calamity to the male. This kind of witchcraft is of two sorts, one temporary and the other permanent. It is called permanent when it lasts up to death and cannot be removed by any natural medicine or other lawful means. It is temporary when it is only to last for a certain time.

Vincent of Beauvais tells the following. At Rome in the time of the Emperor Henry III there was a certain noble and rich young man who had lately married a wife and invited his friends to a sumptuous wedding feast, and they went out after dinner into the fields to play at ball. The bridegroom as leader of the game asked for the ball, and lest his betrothal ring should fall off he put it on the finger of a bronze statue of Venus which was close by, and all turned to the game. He soon grew tired and stopped playing, and came back to the statue to get his ring; but the statue's finger was bent back to the palm of the hand, and however he tried to recover the ring, he could not bend the finger nor draw off the ring. He went back to his friends, but told them nothing about this. In the dark of night he came back with a servant to the statue, and found the finger stretched out as it had been at first, but without the ring. He kept quiet about his loss and went into the house to his newly married wife; and when he entered the bridal chamber and wished to lie with his wife, he felt himself prevented, and something cloudy and dense rolled between his body and his wife's. He could feel this, but he could not see it. By this obstacle he was prevented from embracing his wife; and he also heard a voice saying: 'Live with me, for to-day you have wed me. I am Venus, upon whose finger you placed the ring, which I shall not return.' The man (says S. Antoninus, who takes this story from Vincent of Beauvais) was terrified by such a prodigy, and neither did he dare nor was he able to make any answer, but he spent that night without sleep in deep thought. So it continued for a long time, that whenever he wished to have intercourse with his wife he felt and heard the same thing. In other respects he was healthy, ruled his house well, and was diligent in his military service. At last, driven by his wife's complaints, he took the matter to his parents and they, after due consideration, made it known to a certain suburban priest named Palumbus, who was a necromancer and a master of spells. This man, in return for many fair promises, wrote a letter and gave it to the young man, saying: 'Go at such an hour of the night to the cross-road where four ways meet, and stand there in silent thought. There will go by you the figures of men and women of all ages and conditions, some on horseback and some afoot, some rejoicing and some mourning; but whatever you hear, you must not speak. Following that company will come one of greater stature and bulk sitting on a car, and to him you must silently give the letter to read; and he will at once do what you desire.' The young man did all this exactly as he had been directed, and he saw there among the rest a woman clothed like a harlot riding upon a mule with her hair flowing loose over her shoulders and bound with a golden fillet in front, carrying in her hand a golden rod with which she drove the mule, and appearing almost naked because of the thinness of her garment, and making lascivious gestures. Last came the Lord of the whole rout, bending terrible eyes upon the young man from a superb chariot made of emeralds and pearls, and asked him why he was there. He answered nothing, but held out the letter to him. The demon recognised the seal and, not daring to despise it, read what was written, and thereupon raised his arms to heaven and said: 'Almighty God, how long wilt Thou suffer the iniquities of the priest Palumbus?' He at once sent his servants from his side to wrest the ring from Venus, who after many subterfuges at last yielded it with reluctance. So the young man, having obtained what he sought, at last consummated his long-wished love. But when Palumbus heard of the demon's cry to God about him, he understood that his days were numbered; therefore he himself cut off all his limbs and died in miserable pain, having confessed to unheard of crimes in the presence of the Roman people.

Gotschalcus Hollen, the Augustinian Eremite, writes as follows: . . . I know a woman who wished to cause a divorce between a man and a woman who loved each other, and for this she was to receive payment. She wrote upon some cards two strange characters, together with other devout words, and gave them these cards to wear; yet they did not quarrel. Then she wrote the same words on a cheese which she gave them to eat; and afterwards took a black chicken which she cut in half, and offered one half to the devil with certain sacrificial rites, and gave the other half to the man and woman to eat. After this there arose the greatest hatred between them, so that they could not bear to look at each other. And how did this happen, unless it were a sacrificial offering to the devil? So writes Hollen.

Giovanni Battista Codronchi . . . relates that there was in the town of Sepino, in the Kingdom of Naples, a man named Jacopo whose wife so detested him that, from the very first day of their marriage, they had been so far from being able to consummate the wedding that they could not even live together; and if ever Jacopo tried to approach his wife, she was filled with such fury and rage that she would rather throw herself from the window than submit to him. This was told to a certain religious man to whom they had given hospitality; and he found it difficult to believe the story, and therefore, in order to prove it, asked that the woman should be approached there and then. The husband accordingly hid himself within the house, lest his wife, knowing him to be present, should refuse to come in. The woman came, and being asked the reason for her hatred of her husband began to bemoan her evil fate and said that she could give no reason at all; but she declared that when her husband was absent she was consumed with such a longing and love for him as she could not express in words; but when she went near him to speak to him and look at him, there at once appeared in her imagination such deformed, ugly and horrible monsters in the likeness of her husband that she would rather die than endure him; and that her whole soul and all her strength and part of her life seemed to be drawn into her husband as an evil offering to her own ruin: but when he was again absent she again burned with the same love. The good priest wished to prove the truth of the woman's words and told the women who were with her to bind her by her arms and legs with a strong rope to the bed in the form of a cross; and he told the husband to put off all repugnance and quickly have to do with her. For the priest suspected that the woman might be pretending to be affected in that way so that she might conceal some deformity. The wife, in her desire for her husband, let herself be bound and asked that her husband should be admitted to her: but when he came in, never was seen such terrible fury, no wild beast was ever so fierce or so filled with madness and rage as that woman; for she foamed at the mouth and gnashed her teeth and rolled her eyes, whilst her whole body seemed to be shaken and possessed with demons. The women who were present said that when they touched her belly which was twisting under the ropes, it appeared to be crammed full, and all her skin was covered with weals as if she had been beaten. There was no end to this raging until the husband, tired out with struggling and moved with pity for her, went away.

Cornelius Gemma inquires into the mutation of the feminine into the masculine sex, and the masculine into the feminine, which is admitted by modern physicians to be natural. We read of many women who have become men. Hippocrates writes that at Abdera Phaetula, the wife of Pitheus, had borne him children; but when her husband was sent into exile, after a few months her menstrual courses ceased, and she was smitten with terrible pains all over her body, and acquired the physical features of a man. He says that the same thing happened to Anamisia, the wife of Gorgippus, at Thasos. Livy tells the same story in Book 24 (*de Spoletana muliere*). Pliny says that it is no fable that women are changed into men. Martin Delrio uses the following words (quoting from Pliny, *Historia Naturalis*, VII, 4): 'I myself saw in Africa L. Cossicius, a Tisdritanian citizen, changed into a man on his wedding day.' S. Augustine mentions heathen records of women becoming men, and of hens being changed into the masculine sex, not, however, by witchcraft but naturally: for witches cannot actually do this thing, but only in appearance to deceive us by casting a glamour over our senses with the help of the devil, as we have shown elsewhere.

Giovanni Pontano (*Hist. Neapolit.*) tells that at Gaeta a woman changed into a man after having been married for fourteen years to a fisherman: and another, named Emilia, after having been for twelve years the wife of Antonio Spensa, a citizen of Eboli, dissolved her marriage, married a wife and begot children. He speaks also of another woman who had borne one son to her husband, and suddenly assumed virility, left her husband, and married a woman who bore children to her.

Cocceius Sabellicus has some similar stories which I shall omit, and will set down two instances which occurred in Spain in our own time, and were faithfully described by Antonio de Turrecremata in his *Jardin de las Flores curiosas*.

In the town of Ezgueira in Portugal, about nine leagues from Coimbra, there lived a nobleman who had a daughter named Maria Pacheco. When this girl was at the age when a woman's monthly courses usually begin, instead of a fluid excretion there broke or otherwise grew from those parts a virile member; and so, from being a girl, she suddenly became a pubic young man endowed with virility, and assumed the name of Manoel Pacheco. He then took ship for India and endured much hardship and performed great deeds as a soldier. Returning to his country he married a noble wife: yet Amatus the Portuguese, writing in his *Centuries*, makes no mention of any children, but says that he remained unbearded and with a feminine cast of countenance, these being indications of imperfect virility. Finally Torquemada adds that he heard this from a most trustworthy friend of great authority.

Not far from Benaventana in Spain the wife of a farmer of moderate fortune was ill-treated by her husband because she was barren. Weary of such bad treatment she ran away one night dressed as a man-servant, and in this guise went from place to place earning her living by menial work. After some time, either because of the efficacy of her natural heat or through imagination induced and strengthened by her continuous masculine clothing and work, she found that she had actually turned into a man. Therefore she, who had long been a wife, determined to act the husband, and consummated her marriage with a woman. The secret was kept for a long time, since she did not dare to tell it to any one, until a certain man who had been very well known to her noticed that she was in face very like that farmer's wife who had run away. He asked if he were her brother; whereupon she told him the whole story as it happened, and so it came to light.

Baptista Fergoso (*Exemplorum*, I, 6) writes as follows. At Naples, in the reign of Ferdinand I, Ludovico Guarna, a citizen of Salerno, had five daughters, the two youngest of whom were named Francesca and Carola. When these two girls reached the age of fifteen the genital parts of both of them sprouted into masculinity, so that they changed their clothes and were taken for men, being called Francesco and Carolo.

At Eboli in the same region, a girl had been betrothed for four years. On the first night of her marriage she went to bed with her husband: but either owing to the friction or to some other unknown cause, when the hymen which gave her the appearance of a woman was broken, a male organ stood out. She then went home and sued in the Courts for a return of her dowry, and was thereafter reckoned as a man.

If this can come about naturally, as so many authors maintain, I should think that with God's permission it is possible to the devil, relying upon natural causes.

Almost all the Theologians and learned Philosophers are agreed, and it has been the experience of all times and all nations, that witches practise coition with demons, the men with Succubus devils and the women with Incubus devils. Plato in the *Cratylus*, Philo, Josephus, and the Old Synagogue; S. Cyprian, S. Justin Martyr, Clement of Alexandria, Tertullian, and others have clearly proved that devils can at will fornicate with women. But a more substantial proof is to be found in S. Jerome on *Ephesians* vi, and S. Augustine, . . . who is followed by the consensus of all Theologians, and especially by S. Isidore, chapter 8. The same belief is championed in the Bull of Pope Innocent VIII against witches.

This truth can be proved by argument. For demons can assume the bodies of dead men, or make for themselves out of air a palpable body like that of flesh, and to these they can impart motion and heat at their will. They can therefore create the appearance of sex which is not naturally present, and show themselves to men in a feminine form, and to women in a masculine form, and lie with each accordingly: and they can also produce semen which they have brought from elsewhere, and imitate the natural ejaculation of it.

I add that a child can be born of such copulation with an Incubus devil. To make this clear, it must be known that the devil can collect semen from another place, as from a man's vain dreams, and by his speed and experience of physical laws can preserve that semen in its fertilising warmth, however subtle and airy and volatile it be, and inject it into a woman's womb at the moment when she is most disposed to conceive, making it appear to be done in the natural way, and so mingling it with the woman's ova. Yet it is true that the devils cannot, as animals do, procreate children by virtue of their own strength and substance: for neither between themselves have they any propagation of their own kind, nor are they endowed with any semen which can in the least degree prove fertile. And how should they have semen of their own, since semen is a vital part of the corporeal substance, and (according to Symposianus in his *Problems*) a secretion from well-digested food; whereas devils are substances without corporeal bodies? We say, then, that a child can be born from the copulation of an Incubus with a woman, but that the father of such a child is not the demon but that man whose semen the demon has misused. There are countless examples told by many authors (Jornandus, *de rebus Gothicis* and Luitprend) that the Huns were descended from the union of Fauns with Gothic witches. Chieza (*Hist. Peru*, II, 27) writes that in Spanish America a demon named Corocoton lies with women and that there are born children with two horns. The Japanese claim that their Shaka is of the same sort. Nor are there wanting those who place Luther in this class. And not ten years ago a woman was punished in the chief city of Brabant because she had been brought to bed by a demon. . . .

We shall set down certain instances of the activities of Succubus devils, as well as some more of Incubus devils.

Fifteen years ago, at Bamberg, a certain Peter Stumpf was sentenced to death because he had sinned with a Succubus devil for more than twenty-eight years. This devil had given him a girdle which he had only to put on, and it appeared both to himself and others that he was changed into a wolf. He tried to devour two of his daughters-in-law. He lived with his own daughter and her godmother as his wives. This is all vouched for in the Court records, and is memorised in pictures carved in brass which are for sale.

Remy tells an example which he heard from a trustworthy man named Melchiore Errico, taken from the most closely guarded secrets of the Most Serene Duke of Lorraine. 'There was at Hemingen,' says this man, 'while I was watching my Lord's interests in that place, a certain warlock who, when he was asked by the Judge how he had first been led into such wickedness and, especially, by what wiles the devil had seduced him, freely and openly declared as follows: 'I was a common herdsman, and at dawn of day was gathering my herds from their several houses, when of all the girls who let the cattle out of the stables one especially fired my soul with love, and I began to think more of the bed chamber. The girl, having escaped from this danger, gave birth to a monster of utterly loathsome appearance, such as had never before been seen, as it was said; and lest it should be seen and bring disgrace upon her family, the midwives lit a huge fire and quickly burned it.

A little earlier the same author tells of a Succubus devil as follows. In the district of Gareotha in a village not fourteen miles from Aberdeen, a young man of great beauty openly complained before the Bishop of Aberdeen that for many months he had been tormented by a Succubus devil, as they say, more beautiful than any woman that he had ever seen. He said that she came to him by night through locked doors, coaxed and forced him into her embraces, and went away as the dawn began to break, with scarcely any sound; and that he could by no means, though he had tried many, be delivered from so great and foul a madness. The excellent Bishop at once ordered the young man to remove himself to another place, and to apply his mind more than usual to the Christian Religion, with more devout fasting and prayer; and so, following the advice of the venerable Bishop, the young man was after a few days delivered from the Succubus devil.

Many of the followers of Luther and Melancthon maintained that witches went to their Sabbats in imagination only, and that there was some diabolical illusion in the matter, alleging that their bodies had often been found lying at home in their beds and had never moved from them; and they support their contention with that passage in the Life of S. Germanus concerning the women who met together, as it seemed, in a feast, and yet were all the time sleeping at home. It is certain that such women are very often the victims of illusion, but it is not proved that this is always so. But as Michal the wife of David deceived the soldiers of her father Saul by putting an image in David's room, so we say that the devil can and does place a false body in the bed to deceive the husband while a witch has gone to the Sabbat; and in order that the husband may not suspect she is absent, he either causes him to fall into a heavy sleep, or substitutes a likeness of his wife so that the husband on awakening may think that it is indeed his wife.

(pp. 15–47)

7

Pierre De Lancre

Pierre de Lancre was one of the worst torturers in France on whose orders many people perished in south western France. Perhaps more than any other demonologist he dwelt upon the sexual goings on at Sabbats. The extracts illustrating this preoccupation are short because they had to be translated from French and Latin, as there is no English translation of his main treatise *Tableau de l'inconstance des mauvais anges et demons* (1612).

They do not call him demon, but Little Master, or Martinettus or Martinellus . . . .

The Devil pisses into a hole in the ground and makes holy water from his urine, with which the one who says the Mass sprinkles the assistants with a black asparagus . . . .

He takes the new arrival (i.e. the neophyte) to one side in a clump of trees, in order to embrace her after his own fashion and have carnal knowledge of her. From the evil in his heart he tells her to lie on the ground, face downwards, on both hands and feet, kneeling. In no other way can he have intercourse; and in whatever way the president enjoys her, when his member is taken into the neophyte, it is often cold and flaccid, as his whole body often is. First of all he enters her through the natural passage and leaves there semen which is tainted and yellowy, kept over from some act of pollution at night or at other times; then secondly he enters her through the seat of evacuation and so abuses her immoderately . . . .

The neophyte (new arrival) before the meal goes to have intercourse with some man . . . each one takes his lady aside and has carnal knowledge of her. At times there are monstrous excesses and forms of pollution, as one woman changes place with another and one man with another. There are acts of unnatural abuse between women and similarly between men; or a woman has intercourse with a man outside the proper channel in some other part . . . . A man with a she-devil or a

128

woman with a demon experiences no pleasure, but out of fear and obedience agrees to couple . . . .

But at the second meeting the woman herself, the new recruit, is known carnally by the demon who is her companion and attendant, in the same way as she was known before by the president. After this at subsequent meetings she is not known again by a demon, except when there are not enough men for copulation purposes (there are usually more women than men) and the demons act as stand-ins for men, just as it can happen (tho' seldom) that she-devils make the number up when there is a shortage of women. And so it goes on at other meetings, apart from the first two, in the first of which she is known by the president and, after her return to the meeting, by a she-devil. It is possible to find (not often) cases of a man always having intercourse with a she-devil, a sign of terrible wickedness, and similarly there are some women always having a man or demon at all the meetings.

. . . They all roll around in the straw together: on Sunday with succubus Devils or incubus Devils; on Thursday they commit sodomy; on Saturday bestiality; on other days they do it the natural way . . . . the Devil arranges marriages between witches and warlocks. But as soon as they lie together he gets between them and swives with the witches and takes virginity from the girls . . . .

This lascivious operation is not carried out or practised by them [the devils] for the pleasure of it, because being simple spirits they can derive no pleasure from the senses. But they do it only to make men fall into the precipice where they find themselves, which is the damnation by Very Mighty and Very High God . . . .

Iohannes d'Aguerre confessed that the Devil in the form of a he-goat had his member at the back and had intercourse with women shaking it and pushing it into them from the front . . . .

Marie de Marigrane, aged 15, dwelling at Biarritz, says that she often has seen the Devil copulating with an infinity of women, whom he called by their names and surnames; and that it is his custom to copulate with the pretty ones from the front and with the ugly ones from behind . . . .

Margueritte, daughter of Sore, aged between 16 and 17 years testifies that the Devil, whether he takes the form of a man or a he-goat, always has a member like a donkey, having chosen to imitate the animal which is best endowed. It is long and thick like an arm: when he wants to copulate with one of the girls or women he conjures up a bed of hay on which he makes them lie, which does not at all displease them. And he never appears at the Sabbat in any function whatsoever without having his tool outside in good shape and size. This is the opposite of what Boguet says: that the women saw him with a thing not much larger than a finger and thick in proportion. Perhaps the witches of Labourt are better served by the Satan than those of Franche Comte. . . . It appears that this bad Demon has a half and half member: half of flesh and half of iron, right along; and the same is true of his testicles . . . .

8

George Sinclair

George Sinclair became obsessed with witches' evildoings after his daughters died of an illness. His book *Satan's Invisible World Discovered* (1685) consists of stories about how witches make people ill, mostly reproduced from other writers. Here is an example from pp. 164–5 of the reprint published by Paesons Scholars' Facsimiles (Gainsville, Florida: 1969):

RELATION XXVI.

A Wonderful and Strange Accident which fell out at *Lions* in *France*.

A Lieutenent *of a* Guard *called* Jaquette *having supped one Night in a rich Merchants house, was passing home and by the way, said, I wonder what I have eaten and drunken at the Merchants house, for I find my self so hot, that if I met with the Devils* Dame *this night,* I could not forbear using of her. *Hereupon, a little after, he overtook a young* Gentlewoman *masked, whom he would needs usher home to her Lodging, but discharged all his Company except two. She brought him as to his apprehension, to a little low house hard by the City wall where there were only two* Rooms. *After he had enjoyed her he desired that according to the custom of* French Gentlemen, *his two Comerads might partake also of the same Pleasure. So she admitted them, one after the other. And when all was done, as they sat together, she told them,* if they knew well, who she was none of them would have adventured upon her. *Thereupon she whistled three times, and all evanished. The next morning, the two Comerads, that had gone with the* Lieutenent Jaquette *were found dead under the* City-wall, *among the* Odure and Excrements, *and* Jaquette *himself a little way off half dead, who was taken up and coming to himself again confessed all this, and presently dyed. This may verify the preceeding Relation.*

9

Lodovico Sinistrari

Lodovico Maria Sinistrari – a Franciscan monk, professor of the University of Pavia and a famous theologian – wrote *De Daemonialitate* during the last years of his life (1622–1701) when the wave of persecution had already receded. Though equally preoccupied with the question of sexual temptation, he is much less worried about disease and shows no signs of the obsessional fear of the devil and witches, which is so conspicuous in the writings of the earlier demonologists. Indeed, in contrast to them he makes the consorting with the incubi and succubi into a rather venial sin, albeit he does not disavow torture and other horrendous practices. What is important from the viewpoint of the explanation is that there is no trace here of any influence of the progress of enlightenment: Sinistrari is just as gullible and superstitious as the earlier demonologists but is less afraid and less bloodthirsty. His translator into English, Montague Summers, writes in his Introduction:

> The thesis which Sinistrari sets forth in detail may be stated as follows: There are in existence on earth rational creatures besides man, endowed like him with a body and a soul; they are born and die like him; they are redeemed by Our Lord Jesus Christ, and therefore are capable of being saved or being lost. These rational creatures or animals are swayed by the same emotions and passions, jealousies and lusts, as man. They are affected by material substances; therefore they participate in the matter of those substances, that is to say, they have corporeity. But this corporeity is far more tenuous and subtle than the body of a man. It enjoys a certain rarity, permeability, volatility, and power of sublimation. These creatures are able at will to withdraw themselves from the sight of man.
>
> Charles-René Billuart, the celebrated Dominican (1685–1757), in his *Tractatus de Angelis* expressly declares: 'The same evil spirit may serve as a succubus to a man, and as an incubus to a woman.' So, in general acceptance, the Incubus is a demon, and

more precisely a demon employed for the purpose of fornicating with witches.

Now the Incubus, as Sinistrari uses the term, and as in studying his treatise we must understand it, is not a demon, but he is a *lutin* – there seems to be no exact English term to express him as Sinistrari conceives him. He is frequently mischievous and vexatious; not unseldom rampant and lickerish; a whoremaster, neighing after copulation; but not demoniacal.

The following extracts are taken from *Demoniality*, translated from the Latin and edited by Rev. Montague Summers (London: The Fortune Press, 1927).

DEMONIALITY

The first author who, so far as I know, uses the word *Demoniality* is Juan Caramuel, in his *Fundamental Theology*, and before him I can find no one who distinguishes that crime from *Bestiality*. Indeed, all Moral Theologians, following S. Thomas (II. 2, quest. 154), include, under the specific title of *Bestiality*, '*every kind of carnal intercourse with any thing whatsoever of a different species*': such are the words used by S. Thomas. Cajetan, for instance, in his commentary on that Question, classes intercourse with the Demon under the description of Bestiality; so does Silvester, *de Luxuria*; Bonacina, *de Matrimonio*, quest. 4; and others.

However, it is clear that in the above passage S. Thomas did not allude to intercourse with the Demon. And as shall be demonstrated further on, that intercourse cannot be included in the particular and peculiar species *Bestiality*; and, in order to make that sentence of the holy Doctor tally with truth, it must be admitted that when saying of unnatural sin, '*that committed through intercourse with a thing of different species, it takes the name of Bestiality*,' S. Thomas, by *a thing of different species*, means a living animal, of another species than man: for he could not here use the word *thing* in its most general sense, to mean indiscriminately an animate or inanimate being. In fact, if a man should fornicate with a dead body, he would have to do with a thing of a species quite different from his own (especially according to the Thomists, who deny the form of human corporeity in a corpse); similarly if he were to have connexion with a dead animal: yet, such copulation would not be bestiality, but pollution. What therefore S. Thomas intended here to specify so exactly is carnal intercourse with a living thing of a species different from man, that is to say, with an animal, and he assuredly intends no reference to intercourse with the Demon.

Therefore, connexion with the Demon, whether Incubus or Succubus (which is, properly speaking, *Demoniality*), differs in kind from Bestiality, and does not in conjunction with it form one particular species, as Cajetan wrongly maintains; for, whatever may have been said to the contrary by some early authorities, and later by Caramuel in his *Fundamental Theology*, by Vincenzo Filliucci, and others, unnatural sins differ from each other most distinctly. Such at least is the general doctrine and the contrary opinion has been condemned by Alexander VII. (No. XXIV. of the condemned propositions): first, because each of those sins carries with itself its peculiar and distinct turpitude, opposed to chastity and to human procreation; secondly, because the commission thereof entails each time the sacrifice of some good by reason of the nature attached to the institution of the venereal act, the normal end of which is human generation; lastly, because each has a different motive, which in itself is sufficient to bring about, in divers and several ways, the deprivation of the same good, as has been clearly shown by Filliucci, Crespinus, and Caramuel.

It follows that Demoniality differs in kind from Bestiality, for each has its peculiar and distinct turpitude, opposed to chastity and human procreation. Bestiality is connexion with a living beast, endowed with its own proper senses and impulses; Demoniality, on the contrary, is copulation with a corpse (in accordance at least with the general opinion which shall be considered hereafter), a senseless and motionless corpse which is but accidentally moved through the power of the Demon. Now, if fornication with the dead body of a man, or a woman, or a beast differ in kind from Sodomy and Bestiality, there is the same difference with regard to *Demoniality*, which, according to the general opinion, is the intercourse of man with a dead body accidentally endued with motion.

Another proof follows: in sins against nature, the unnatural semination (which cannot be regularly followed by procreation) is a genus; but the object of such semination is the difference which marks the species under the genus. Thus, whether semination takes place on the ground, or on an inanimate body, it is pollution; if with a male *in uase præpostero*, it is Sodomy

(*Sodomia perfecta*); with a beast, Bestiality: crimes which unquestionably all differ from each other in species, just as the ground,
the corpse, the man and the beast, passive objects of such
emission of semen, differ in species from each other. But the
difference betwen the Demon and the beast is not only specific,
it is more than specific: the nature of the one is corporeal, of the
other incorporeal, which makes a generic difference. Whence it
follows that several emissions of semen practised on different
objects differ in species from each other: and that is, according
to the intention of the act.

. . . it is acknowledged by all Moral Theologians that carnal
connexion with the Devil, or a familiar, is much more heinous
than the same act committed with any beast whatsoever. Now,
in the same particular and peculiar species of sins, one sin is not
more heinous than another; all are equally grave: it is the same
whether connexion is had with a bitch, an ass, or a mare; whence
it follows that if *Demoniality* is more heinous than Bestiality,
those two acts are not of the same species. And let it not be
argued . . . that *Demoniality* is always more heinous on account
of the offence to religion from the worship rendered to the
Demon or the compact of fellowship entered into with him: since
it has been shown above, that these circumstances do not
always occur in the connexion of man with Incubi and Succubi;
moreover, if in the genus of unnatural sin *Demoniality* is more
grievous than Bestiality, the offence to Religion is quite foreign
to that aggravation, and accidental, since it is foreign to that
genus itself.

Therefore, having laid down the specific difference between
Demoniality and Bestiality, so that the gravity thereof may be
duly appreciated in view of the penalty to be inflicted (and that
is our most essential object), we must needs inquire in how
many different ways the sin of *Demoniality* may be committed.
There is no lack of people who, mightily proud of their small
stock of knowledge, venture to deny what has been written by
the gravest authors and what is, moreover, testified by every
day experience: namely, that the Demon, whether Incubus or
Succubus, unites carnally not only with men and women, but
also with beasts. They allege that it all proceeds from the human
imagination troubled by the craft of the Demon, and that it is
nothing but phantasmagoria, glamour, and diabolical spells. The
like happens, they say, to Witches who, under the influence of

an illusion brought on by the Demon, imagine that they attend the nightly sports, dances, revels and sabbats, and there have carnal intercourse with the Demon, though in reality they are not bodily transferred to those places nor do they take any part in these abominations. But the reality and the truth of all this have been explicitly laid down by Episcopal Capitularies, by the Council of Ancyra, by the Roman synods under Pope S. Damascus I. These are cited by Lorinus of Avignon.

Of course, there is no question that sometimes young women, deceived by the Demon, imagine they are actually taking part, in their flesh and blood, in the sabbats of Witches, and all this is merest fantasy. Thus, in a dream, one sometimes fancies that one is sleeping with someone else, and there is an emission of semen, yet that connexion is wholly unreal and imaginary, and often brought about by a diabolical illusion: and here the above-mentioned Episcopal Capitularies and Councils are perfectly right. But this is not always the case; on the contrary, it more often happens that Witches are bodily present at sabbats and have an actual carnal and corporeal connexion with the Demon, and that likewise Wizards copulate with the Succubus or female Demon. Such is the opinion of Theologians as well as of jurists, many of whose names will be found at length in the *Compendium Maleficarum*, or *Chronicle of Witches*, by Fra Francesco Maria Guazzo. It is maintained by Grilland, Remy, S. Peter Damian, Silvester, Alfonso à Castro, Cajetan, Père Pierre Crespet, Bartolomeo Spina, Giovanni Lorenzo Anania. This doctrine is also therein confirmed by eighteen actual instances adduced from the recitals of learned and truthful men whose testimony is beyond suspicion, and which prove that Wizards and Witches are indeed bodily present at sabbats and most shamefully copulate with Demons, Incubi or Succubi. And, after all, to settle the question, we have the authority of S. Augustine, who, speaking of carnal intercourse between men and the Demon, expresses himself as follows, book xvth, chap. 23rd, of the *City of God*: '*It is widely credited, and such belief is confirmed by the direct or indirect testimony of thoroughly trustworthy people, that Sylvans and Fauns, commonly called Incubi, have frequently molested women, sought and obtained from them coition. There are even Demons, whom the Gauls call Duses or Boggarts, who very regularly indulge in those unclean practices: the fact is testified by so many and such weighty authorities, that it were impudent to doubt it.*' Such are the very words of S. Augustine.

Now, several authors assert, and it is confirmed by numerous experiments, that the Demon has two ways of copulating carnally with men or women: the one which he uses with Witches or Wizards, the other with men or women who know nothing of witchcraft.

In the first case, the Demon does not copulate with Witches or Wizards until after a solemn profession, in virtue of which such wretched creatures yield themselves up to him . . . the Demon imprints on them some mark, especially on those whose constancy he suspects. That mark, moreover, is not always of the same shape or figure: sometimes it is the likeness of a hare, sometimes a toad's foot, sometimes a spider, a puppy, a dormouse. It is imprinted on the most hidden parts of the body: with men, under the eyelids, or it may be under the armpits, or on the lips, on the shoulder, the fundament, or somewhere else; with women, it is usually on the breasts or the privy parts. Now, the stamp which imprints those marks is none other but the Devil's claw. When all these rites have been performed in accordance with the instructions of the mystagogues who initiate the novices, these then promise never to worship the Blessed Sacrament; to insult all Saints and especially the most Holy Mother of God; to trample under foot and defile Holy Images, the Cross, and the Relics of Saints; never to use the sacraments or sacramentals; never to make a good confession to the priest, but to keep always hidden from him their intercourse with the Demon. The Demon, in exchange, engages to give them always prompt assistance; to fulfil their desires in this world and to make them happy after their death. The solemn profession being thus made, each has assigned to himself a Devil called *Magistellus* or Little Master, with whom he retires aside for carnal satisfaction; the said Devil assuming the shape of a woman if the initiated person be a man, the shape of a man, sometimes of a satyr, sometimes a buck-goat, if it be a woman who has been received a witch. Guazzo; *loc. cit.*

If we seek to learn from these Authorities how it is possible that the Demon, who has no body, yet can perform actual coitus with man or woman, they unanimously answer that the Demon assumes the corpse of another human being, male or female as the case may be, or that, from the mixture of other materials, he shapes for himself a body endowed with motion, by means of which body he copulates with the human being; and they add that when women are desirous of becoming pregnant by the Demon (which occurs only with the consent and at the express wish of the said women), the Demon is transformed into a Succubus, and during the act of coition with some man receives therefrom human semen; or else he procures pollution from a man during his sleep, and then he preserves the spilt semen at its natural heat, conserving it with the vital essence. This, when he has connexion with the woman, he introduces into her womb, whence follows impregnation. Such is the teaching of Guazzo, book I, ch. 12, and he proves it by a number of quotations and instances taken from many learned Doctors.

At other times also the Demon, whether Incubus or Succubus, copulates with men or women from whom, however, he receives none of the sacrifices, homage or offerings which he is wont to exact from Wizards or Witches, as aforesaid. He is then but a passionate lover, having only one desire; the carnal possession of those whom his lust craves. Of this there are numerous instances to be found in authors of no small repute, amongst whom we read of the case of Menippus Lycius, who long cohabited with a woman, and when she had served him sexually many times and oft, so doted on her that she persuaded him to marry her; but a certain philosopher, who happened to be present at the wedding banquet, having guessed what the woman was, told Menippus that he had to deal with a *Compusa*, that is a Succubus; whereupon the bride vanished shrieking and wailing bitterly.

Hector Boece . . . also relates the adventure of a young Scotchman, who, during many months, although the doors and windows of his chamber were ever fast shut, was visited in his bed-room by a Succubus of the most enchanting beauty; she resorted to every blandishment, caresses, kisses, embraces, entreaties, to prevail upon him to fornicate with her: but she could not succeed with the chaste young man.

We read likewise of numerous women incited to coition by an Incubus, and who, though reluctant at first of yielding to him, are soon moved by his prayers, tears, and endearments; for he is a desperate lover and must not be denied. And although this comes sometimes of the craft of some Wizard who avails himself of the agency of the Demon, yet the Demon not infrequently acts thus on his own account, as Guazzo informs us, *Compendium*

Maleficarum, III. 8; and this happens not only with women, but also with mares; for if they readily comply with his desire, he pets them, and plaits their manes in elaborate and inextricably reticulated tresses; but if they resist, he ill-treats and strikes them, infects them with the glanders and lampass, and may finally kill them, as is shown by daily experience.

Taking for granted the truth of the recitals concerning the intercourse of Incubi and Succubi with men and beasts, recitals so numerous that it would be sheer impudence to deny the fact, as is said by S. Augustine, whose testimony is given above (No. 10) (*City of God*, XV. 23), I argue: Where the peculiar passion of the sense is found, there also, of necessity, is the sense itself: for, according to the principles of philosophy, the peculiar passion flows from nature, that is to say that, where the acts and operations of the sense are found, there also is the sense, the operations and acts being but its external form. Now, those Incubi and Succubi present acts, operations, peculiar passions, which spring from the senses; they are therefore endowed with senses. But senses cannot exist without concomitant component organs, without a combination of soul and body. Incubi and Succubi have therefore body and soul, and, consequentially, are animals; but their acts and operations are also those of a rational soul; their soul is therefore rational; and thus, from first to last, they are rational animals.

The appetitive desire of coition is a sensual desire; the grief, sadness, wrath, rage, occasioned by the denial of coition, are sensual passions, as is seen with all animals; generation through coition is evidently a sensual operation. Now, all that happens with Incubi, as has been shown above: they incite women, sometimes even men; if denied, they sadden and storm, like lovers: *amantes, amentes*; they practise perfect coition, and sometimes beget. It must therefore be inferred that they have senses, and consequently a body; consequently also, that they are perfect animals. More than that: in spite of closed doors and windows they enter wherever they please; their body is therefore slender: they foreknow and foretell the future, compose and divide, all which operations are proper to a rational soul; they therefore possess a rational soul and are, in fine, rational animals.

Doctors generally reply that it is the Evil Spirit that perpetrates those impure acts, simulates passions, love, grief at the denial of coition, in order to entice souls to sin and to undo them; and that, if he copulates and begets, it is with assumed sperm and a body not truly his own, as aforesaid (No. 24).

But then, there are Incubi that have connexion with horses, mares and other beasts, and, as shown by everyday experience, ill-treat them if they are averse to coition; yet, in those cases, it can no longer be adduced that the Demon simulates the appetite for coition in order to bring about the ruin of souls, since beasts are not capable of everlasting damnation. Besides, love and wrath with them are productive of quite opposite effects. For, if the loved woman or beast humours them, those Incubi behave very well; on the contrary, they use them most savagely when irritated and enraged by a denial of coition: this is amply proved by daily experience: those Incubi therefore have truly sexual passions and desires. Besides, the Evil Spirits, the incorporeal Demons who copulate with Sorceresses and Witches, constrain them to Demon worship, to the abjuration of the Catholic Faith, to the commission of enchantments, magic, and foul crimes, as preliminary conditions to the infamous intercourse, as has been above stated. . . . now, Incubi endeavour nothing of the kind: they are therefore not Evil spirits.

. . . The Evil Spirits . . . possess bodies or, through sheer malice, infect them with diseases and other infirmities; [Incubi] . . . neither possess bodies nor infect them with diseases; they, at most, annoy them by blows and ill-treatment. If they cause the mares to grow lean because of their not yielding to coition, it is merely by taking away their provender, in consequence of which they fall off and finally die. To that purpose the Incubus need not use a natural agent, as the Evil Spirit does when imparting a disease: it is enough that he should exert his own native organic force. Likewise, when the Evil Spirit possesses bodies and infects them with diseases, it is most frequently through signs agreed upon with himself, and arranged by a witch or a wizard, which signs are usually natural objects, indued with their own noxious virtue, and, of course, opposed by other equally natural objects endowed with a contrary virtue. But not so the Incubus: it is of his own accord, and without the co-operation of either witch or wizard, that he pursues his molestation. Besides, the natural things which put the Incubi to flight exert their virtue and bring about a result without the intervention of any exorcism or blessing; it cannot therefore be said that the ejection of the Incubus is initiated by natural, and completed by divine virtue, since there is in this case no particular invocation of the divine Name, but the mere effect of a natural object, in which God co-operates only as the universal agent, the author of nature, the first of efficient causes.

To illustrate this important point, I will here relate two stories, the first of which I have from a good confessor of Nuns, a man of integrity and fair repute, and most worthy of credit; the second I was eye-witness to myself.

In a certain convent of holy Nuns there resided, as a boarder, a young maiden of noble family, who was tempted by an Incubus that appeared to her both by day and by night, and with the most earnest entreaties, the prayers of a passionate lover crazed for love, incessantly besought her to lie with him; but she, supported by the grace of God and the frequent use of the sacraments, stoutly resisted the temptation. Yet, notwithstanding all her devotions, fasts and vows, maugre the exorcisms, the blessings, the injunctions showered by exorcists on the Incubus that he should desist from molesting her; in spite of the vast number of Relics and other holy objects collected in the maiden's room, of the lighted candles kept burning there all night, the Incubus none the less persisted in appearing to her constantly, in the shape of an exceptionally handsome young man. At last, among other learned men, whose advice had been taken on the subject, was a very profound Theologian who, observing that the maiden was of a thoroughly phlegmatic temperament, surmised that that Incubus was an aqueous Demon (there are in fact, as is testifed by Guazzo (*Compendium Maleficarum*, I. 19), igneous, aerial, phlegmatic, earthly, and subterranean demons who avoid the light of day), and so he prescribed a continual suffumigation in the room. A new vessel, made of earthenware and glass, was accordingly introduced, and filled with sweet calamus, cubeb seed, roots of both aristolochies, great and small cardamom, ginger, long-pepper, caryophylleæ, cinnamon, cloves, mace, nutmegs, calamite storax, benzoin, aloes-wood and roots, one ounce of fragrant sandal, and three quarts of half brandy and water; the vessel was then set on hot ashes in order to force forth and upwards the fumigating vapour, and the cell was kept closed. As soon as the suffumigation was done, the Incubus came, but never dared enter the cell; only, if the maiden left it for a walk in the garden or the cloister, he appeared to her, though invisible to others, and throwing his arms round her neck, stole or rather snatched kisses from her, to her intense disgust. At last, after a new consultation, the Theologian prescribed that she should carry about her person pills and pomanders made of the most exquisite perfumes, such as musk, amber, civet, Peruvian balsam, and other essences. Thus furnished, she went for a walk in the garden, where the Incubus suddenly appeared to her with a threatening face, and in a black rage. He did not approach her, however, but, after biting his finger as if meditating revenge, suddenly disappeared and was never more seen by her.

Here is the other story. In the great Carthusian monastery of Pavia there lived a Deacon, Augustine by name, who was subjected by a certain Demon to excessive, unheard-of, and scarcely credible vexations. Many exorcists made repeated endeavours to secure his riddance, yet all spiritual remedies had proved unavailing. I was consulted by the Vicar of the convent, who had the care of the unfortunate cleric. Seeing the inefficacy of all customary exorcisms, and remembering the above-related instance, I advised a suffumigation similar to the one that has been detailed, and prescribed that the young Deacon should carry about his person fragrant pills and comfits of the same kind; moreover, as he was in the habit of using snuff, and was very fond of brandy, I advised snuff and brandy perfumed with musk. The Demon appeared to him by day and by night, under various shapes, as a skeleton, a pig, an ass, an Angel, a bird; with the figure of one or other of the monks, once even with that of his own Superior the Prior, exhorting him to keep his conscience clean, to trust in God, to confess frequently; he persuaded him to let him hear his sacramental confession, recited with him the psalms *Exsurgat Deus* and *Qui habitat*, and the Gospel according to S. John: and when they came to the words *Uerbum caro factum est*, he genuflected devoutly, then donning a stole which was in the cell, and taking the aspergillum, he blessed with holy water the cell and the bed, and, as if he had really been the Prior, enjoined on the Demon not to venture in future to molest his subordinate; he next incontinently disappeared, thus betraying what he was, for otherwise the young Deacon would have taken him for his Prior. Now, notwithstanding the suffumigations and perfumes I had prescribed, the Demon did not desist from his wonted apparitions; more than that, assuming the features of his victim, he went to the Vicar's room, and asked for some snuff and brandy perfumed with musk, of which, he said, he was extremely fond. Having received both, he vanished in the twinkling of an eye, thus showing the Vicar that he had been mocked by the Demon; and this was amply confirmed by the Deacon, who affirmed upon his oath that he had not gone that day to the Vicar's cell. When these circumstances were told to me, I inferred that, far from being aqueous like the Incubus who was in love with the maiden above spoken of, this Demon was igneous, or, at the very least, aerial, since he delighted in hot substances such as warm vapours, perfumes, snuff and brandy. My surmises were greatly confirmed by the temperament of the young Deacon, which was choleric and sanguine, choler, however, somewhat predominating; for these Demons never approach any save those whose temperament tallies with their own. And this is another confirmation of my views regarding their corporeity. I therefore advised the Vicar to let the junior monk take herbs that are cold by nature, such as water-lily, agrimony, spurge, mandrake, house-leek, plantain, henbane, and others of a similar family, knit two little bundles of them and hang them up, one at his window, the other at the door of his cell, taking care to strow some also on the floor and on the bed. Marvellous to say! the Demon appeared again, but remained outside the room, which he would not enter; and, on the Deacon inquiring of him his motives for such unwonted reserve, he burst out into invectives against me for giving such advice, disappeared, and never returned thither again.

Before the Flood, when the air was not yet so thick, Demons came upon earth and had intercourse with women, thus procreating Giants whose stature was nearly equal to that of the Demons, their fathers. But now it is not so: the Incubi who approach women are aqueous and of small stature; that is why they appear in the shape of little men, and, being aqueous, they are most lecherous. Lust and damp go together: Poets have depicted Venus as born of the sea, in order to show, as is explained by Mythologists, that lust takes its source in damp. When, therefore, Demons of short stature impregnate women nowadays, the children that are born are not giants, but men of ordinary size. It should, moreover, be known that when Demons have carnal intercourse with women in their own natural body, without having recourse to any disguise or artifice, the women do not see them, or if they do, see but an almost doubtful, vague, barely sensible shadow, as was the case with the female we spoke of, . . . who, when embraced by an Incubus, scarcely felt his touch. But, when they want to be seen by their mistresses, and to taste to the full the joys of human copulation, they assume a visible disguise and a palpable body. By what means this is effected, is their secret, which our circumscribed Philosophy is unable to discover. The only thing we know is that such disguise or body could not consist merely in concrete air, since this must take place through condensation, and therefore by the influence of cold; a body thus formed would feel like ice, and in the venereal act could afford women no pleasure, but would give them pain; and it is the reverse that takes place.

The distinction being admitted between wholly spiritual Demons, who have intercourse with witches, and Incubi, who have to do with women that are nowise witches, we must now inquire into the heinousness of the crime in both cases.

The intercourse of witches with Demons, from its accompanying circumstances, apostasy from the Faith, the worship of the Devil, and so many other abominations as related above, . . . is the greatest of all sins which can be committed by man; and, considering the hideous enormity against Religion which is presupposed by coition with the Devil, Demoniality is assuredly the most grievous of all carnal offences. But, taking the sins of the flesh as such, exclusive of the sins against Religion, Demoniality should be reduced to simple pollution. The reason, a most convincing one, is that the Devil who swives a witch is a pure spirit, has reached the goal and is damned, as has been said above; if, therefore, he copulates with witches, it is in a body assumed or made by himself, according to the common opinion of Theologians. Though set in motion, that body is not a living one; and it follows that the human being, male or female, who has connexion with such a body, is guilty of the same offence as if he copulated with an inanimate body or a corpse, which would be simple pollution, as we have shown elsewhere. It has, moreover, been truly observed by Cajetan, that such intercourse can very well carry with it the guilt of other crimes, according to the body assumed by the Devil, and the member used: thus, if he should assume the body of a kinswoman, or of a nun, such a crime would be incest or sacrilege; if coition took place in the shape of a beast, or *in uase præpostero*, it would be Bestiality or Sodomy.

As for intercourse with an Incubus, wherein is to be found no element, no, not even the least, of offence against Religion, it is hard to discover a reason why it should be more grievous than Bestiality and Sodomy. For, as we have said above, if Bestiality is more grievous than Sodomy, it is because man degrades the dignity of his kind by mixing with a beast, of a kind much inferior to his own. But, when copulating with an Incubus, it is quite the reverse: for the Incubus, by reason of his rational and immortal spirit, is equal to man; and, by reason of his body, more noble because more subtile, so he is more perfect and more dignified than man. Consequently, when having intercourse with an Incubus, man does not degrade, but rather dignifies, his nature; and, taking that into consideration, Demoniality cannot be more grievous than Bestiality.

It is, however, commonly held to be more grievous, and the reason I take to be this: that it is a sin against Religion to hold any communication with the Devil, either with or without a compact, for instance by habitually or familiarly companying with him, by asking his assistance, counsel or favour, or by seeking from him the revelation of things to be, the knowledge of the past, of absent things, or of circumstances otherwise hidden. Thus, men and women, by mixing with Incubi, whom they do not know to be animals but believe to be devils, sin through intention, *ex conscientia erronea*, and their sin is in intention the same, when having intercourse with Incubi, as if such intercourse took place with devils; wherefore the guilt of their crime is exactly the same.

SUMMARY

1. *Distinctions to be made in the proof of the crime of Demoniality.*
2. *Signs proving the intercourse of a Witch with the Devil.*
3. *The frank confession of the Sorcerer himself is requisite for a full conviction.*
4. *Tale of a Nun who copulated with an Incubus.*
5. *If the indictment is supported by the recitals of eye-witnesses, torture may be resorted to and employed.*

1. As regards the proof of that crime, a distinction must be

made of the kind of Demoniality, to wit: whether it is that which is practised by Witches or Wizards with the Devil, or that which other persons perform with Incubi.

2. In the first case, the compact entered into with the Devil being proved, the evidence of *Demoniality* follows as a necessary consequence; for, the purpose, both of Witches and Wizards, in the midnight sabbats that take place, after feasting and dancing, is none other but that infamous intercourse; moreover there can be no witness of that crime, since the Devil, visible to the Witch, escapes the sight of all beside. Sometimes, it is true, women have been seen in the woods, in the fields, in groves and dingles, lying on their backs, naked to their very navels, in the posture of venery, all their limbs quivering with the orgastic spasm, as is noted by Guazzo . . . . In such a case there would be a very strong suspicion of this crime, particularly if supported by other signs; and I am inclined to believe that such a circumstance, sufficiently proved by good witnesses, would justify the Judge in resorting to torture in order to ascertain the truth; especially if, shortly after that action, a sort of black smoke had been seen to issue from the woman, and she had been noticed to rise, as is also noted by Guazzo; for it might be inferred that that smoke or shadow had been the Devil himself, fornicating with the woman. Likewise if, as has more than once happened, according to the same author, a woman had been seen to fornicate with a mysterious stranger, who, when the action was over, suddenly disappeared.

3. Again, in order to prove conclusively that a person is a Wizard or a Witch, the actual confession of such person is requisite: for there can be no witnesses to the fact, unless perhaps other Sorcerers giving evidence at the trial against their accomplices; and from their being confederates in the crime, their statement is not conclusive and does not justify the recourse to torture, should not other indications be forthcoming, such as the seal of the Devil stamped on their body . . . or the finding in their dwelling, after a search, of signs and instruments of the diabolic art: for example, bones and especially, a skull, hair artfully plaited, intricate knots of feathers, wings, feet or skeletons of bats, toads, or serpents, unfamiliar and, perhaps, noxious seeds, wax figures, vessels filled with unknown powder, oil or viscid ointments, etc., as are usually detected by Judges who, upon a charge being brought against Sorcerers, proceed to their apprehension and the search of their houses.

4. The proof of copulation with an Incubus offers the same difficulty; for, no less than other Demons, the Incubus is, at will, invisible to all but his mistress. Yet, it has not seldom happened that Incubi have allowed themselves to be surprised in the act of carnal intercourse with women, now in one shape, now in another.

In a certain Convent (I mention neither its name nor that of the town where it is situate, so as not to recall to memory a past scandal), there was a Nun, who, as is usual with women and especially with nuns, had quarrelled about some silly trifles with one of her sister-nuns, the occupant of the cell adjoining hers. Quick at observing all the doings of this religious with whom she was at loggerheads, our neighbour noticed that, several days in succession, instead of walking with her companions in the garden after dinner she retired to her cell, where she locked herself in with unwonted precautions. Curious to know what she could be doing there all that time, the inquisitive Nun betook herself to her own cell. Presently she heard a sound, as of two voices conversing in subdued tones (which she could easily do, since the two cells were divided but by a slight partition), then a certain noise, the creaking of a bed, groans and sighs, as of two lovers in an orgasm of love. Her wonderment was now raised to the highest pitch, and she redoubled her attention in order to ascertain who was in the cell. But when, three times running, she had seen no other nun come out save her rival, she strongly suspected that a man had been secretly introduced and was kept hidden there. She went accordingly and reported the whole thing to the Abbess, who, after taking counsel with the Discreets, resolved that she would herself listen to the sounds and observe the strange happenings which had been thus denounced to her, so as to avoid any hasty or inconsiderate act. In consequence, the Abbess and her confidents repaired to the cell of the informer, and thence heard the voices and other noises that had been described. Inquiry was made to ascertain whether any of the Nuns could be shut in with this other one; and when this was found not to be the case, the Abbess and her attendants went to the door of the closed cell, and knocked repeatedly, but to no purpose: the Nun neither answered, nor opened. The Abbess threatend to have the door broken in, and even ordered a lay-sister to force it with a crow-bar. The Nun then opened her door: a search was made and no one found. Being asked with whom she had been talking, and the why and wherefore of the bed creaking, of the long-drawn sighs, etc., she denied everything.

But, since matters went on just the same as before, the rival Nun, becoming slyer and more inquisitive than ever, contrived to bore a hole through the partition, so as to be able to discover exactly what was happening inside the cell; and what should she espy but a comely youth lying with the Nun, a sight she took good care to let the others enjoy by the same means. An accusation was soon laid before the Bishop: the guilty Nun still endeavoured to deny all; but at last, threatened with the torture, she confessed to having been long indecently intimate with an Incubus.

5. When, therefore, indications are forthcoming, such as those detailed above, a charge might be brought after a searching inquiry; yet, without the confession of the accused, the offence should not be regarded as fully proven, even if the intercourse were actually beheld by eye-witnesses; for it sometimes happens that, in order utterly to undo an innocent female, the Devil feigns such intercourse by means of some glamour or delusion. In those cases, the Ecclesiastical Judge therefore must trust but to his own eyes alone.

(pp. 1–5, 6–8, 10–13, 49–59, 85–9, 93–7)

Appendix One

The Impact of Aids on Social Life: Possibilities and Likelihoods

PRELIMINARY REMARKS

According to a report published in *Doctor*, June 1987, 791 cases of Aids have been reported in the United Kingdom by May 1987, which was 431 more than a year previously. This gives a rate which is well above doubling every year. But let us extrapolate the trend on the conservative assumption that the number only doubles itself every year. This results in 101,248 sufferers (not mere carriers) in 1995, 1,619,968 in 1999 and 51,838,976 in 2004. Before the end of the year everybody would be sick and the population would become extinct in 2005.

Fortunately there are good reasons for being confident that this will not happen and that this island will still be inhabited in twenty years' time. Extrapolations must not be taken as predictions. Often their purpose is to show that the present trend will be reversed in one way or another, because it is leading to a situation which we know to be impossible. It has been calculated for example that if the production of goods continued to grow at the nineteen-seventies rate, then within a few centuries the yearly output would surpass the total mass of the globe. Or if the world's population continued to grow at its present rate, then within a millenium the diameter of the human mass would be expanding at the speed of light. In contrast to these eventualities, the extinction of a species is a perfectly possible event which has happened many times.

Being lethal and incurable but not immediately disabling, Aids is capable of exterminating mankind. Its spread may be arrested but (barring some miraculous twist in the evolution of the virus) that can happen only in consequence of an adaptation to the new situation. Such an adaptation can occur only under certain conditions and must have far-reaching consequences. To explore these is the purpose of this Appendix.

Reactions to a calamity may be adaptive or non-adaptive. Some of the latter may even aggravate the situation, as when a panic causes a stampede. In the present context I call adaptive the reactions which tend to contain the infection, and non-adaptive those which produce no such effect. Applying this distinction to history, we can view puritanism as (at least to a large extent) an adaptive reaction to the arrival of syphilis, whereas the witch hunts were clearly non-adaptive. By fostering premarital chastity and marital fidelity, puritanism helped its followers to survive and prosper in the midst of the epidemic. The abolition of the practice of absolving sins after a confession may have contributed to this effect by adding a deterrent: the ineffaceability of sin corresponded to the incurability of syphilitic infection. The introduction of divorce (with financial, moral and even legal penalties for adultery), as well as the abolition of celibacy of the clergy, seem to have made illicit copulation somewhat less common, while the dissolution of the monastic orders may have reduced homosexual practices as well as fornication.

In contrast, nothing of this kind could have been achieved by the witch hunts. They might perhaps have helped to contain the epidemic had they been directed against syphilitics. But the bias against women is a sufficient proof that this was not so because there is not the slightest reason to suppose that there were more syphilitic women than men. Although prostitutes and flagrant fornicators of low status ran a greater risk of being picked upon, there is no evidence of any systematic concentration on them.

One aspect of puritanism which was not obviously adaptive was the avoidance of speaking about sexual acts or parts. Nevertheless it might have constituted an obstacle to fornication by helping to maintain the atmosphere of horror around carnal indulgence. On the other hand, however, it fostered ignorance which in some ways may have facilitated infection. The reaction of most governments and public bodies to the danger of Aids contrasts with this feature of puritanism. Nobody would have thought it possible thirty years ago that government handouts would make plain references to practices which were until recently regarded as abominable and unmentionable perversions, or that condoms would not only be advertised but also recommended. The concept of the obscene has been made also obsolescent by the campaigns to promote 'safe sex' by appealing to fear.

Bearing in mind the aforementioned distinction, let us look first at the possible changes which can be regarded as adaptive.

MODES OF ADAPTATION

The course of an epidemic is determined by the interplay of the following factors:

(1) Changes in the nature of the micro-organism.
(2) Physiological changes in human organisms which affect their resistance either to the initial infection or the development of the illness.
(3) Availability of remedies.
(4) Existence or development of patterns of behaviour which facilitate or impede contagion.

(1) Changes in the nature of the micro-organism

It is conceivable that the HIV virus might change in such a way that it loses its virulence, but there is no reason to expect it. Usually, when a disease becomes less virulent (as has happened with syphilis in the seventeenth century) it is because of changes in the other factors. It is equally possible that the virus becomes transmissible in new ways and, therefore, more virulent. If it became capable of being transmitted like the common cold, mankind would probably become extinct. As there would be no room for sociological predictions in such a case, I shall leave this possibility aside and proceed on the assumption that the Aids virus more or less retains its present nature. I am also assuming that the spread of the disease in the heterosexual population which has happened in Africa can happen elsewhere, as there is no evidence that vulnerability to Aids depends on race.[1] If it is true that Aids originated in Africa, then it is not surprising that it has progressed further there, although special conditions might have made it spread particularly fast. I do not believe, however, that it could have been there a long time because, if we assume that it originated there say sixty years ago, then, at its present rate of spread, it should have already caused great depopulation.

(2) Changes in the human organism

A population can develop resistance to a disease naturally (i.e. without vaccination) in two ways. The first is by individual organisms learning to defend themselves more effectively against the entry of the micro-organism, either by having surmounted the illness or through a process which can be described as natural vaccination: by getting doses of bacteria or viruses which are sufficient to provoke the defence system to counterattack effectively and to prepare itself for future attacks, but not large enough to break through the body's defence and cause an illness.[2] This way of developing resistance is impossible in the case of Aids because this virus attacks the defence system and destroys its ability to function. The other way in which a population can develop resistance against a disease is by selective survival and reproduction: some individuals may have a natural resistance and only they survive to produce the next generation which, therefore, inherits this trait. However, this process of adaptation is possible only if there are some individuals – be they a tiny minority – who are naturally resistant. It is not known whether there are people with natural resistance to Aids. If there are such individuals, the ratio of their number to the total population of the world, would determine how many would have to die before our species could acquire an immunity to Aids. The speed of elimination of the non-resistant type would depend on whether the resistant type can escape infection altogether, or whether they would become carriers who have a permanent resistance against developing the illness. In the latter case they might act as propagators of the disease, whose presence accelerates the dying out of non-resistant types.

Although it is not known whether there are people with natural immunity, it is certain that there are many – probably the great majority – who do not have it. It follows that a natural adaptation – if possible at all – would entail massive depopulation.

(3) The availability of remedies

A technical adaptation to a new disease can take place through the invention or the new application of a remedy which achieves one of these three goals:

(1)   artificially endows the organism with resistance either by

vaccination or (what might be possible in the future) genetic engineering.

(2) kills the micro-organisms which have entered the body by a chemical substance or some other method such as radiation.

(3) impedes the transfer of micro-organisms from one body to another either by killing them in transit with an antiseptic or by erecting a barrier such as protective clothing, containers, etc.

It is impossible to predict an invention because anyone who could prove rather than guess that an invention will be made, would have to possess the knowledge as to how it could be made, and would therefore have already made it. So, even the specialists at the forefront of relevant research can only hope or expect that they will find a cure for Aids, but hopes and expectations often turn out to be vain. This happens even in technology which deals with much simpler entities than organisms and their interactions. For example, it is already forty years since we have been told that nuclear fusion power was just round the corner. In medicine additional uncertainty is generated by the constant struggle between pharmacology and evolution, as micro-organisms acquire immunity to new medicines and new variants spring up. Mutagenic pollutants, as well as the depletion of the ozone in the stratosphere, are probably raising the frequency of mutations, while ecological changes are creating new niches to be occupied. In any case, medical progress has followed unexpected paths. Nobody imagined a hundred (or even fifty) years ago that artificial insemination or transplantations of organs would become practicable before a cure for arthritis, the common cold or rheumatism was found. It is therefore perfectly possible that no cure for Aids will be found . . . or at least for a very long time.

A permanent amelioration of the general situation can be achieved only through a remedy which acts decisively either by endowing the organisms with immunity or by exterminating the virus. A medicament like the one presently available, which merely suppresses (or only delays) the development of the illness without getting rid of the infection, may help the patient but at the risk of aggravating the collective situation by enabling the carrier to go on infecting others, unless it 'helps' him only to the point of prolonging his agony. There is also a possibility (the likelihood of which I cannot judge) that ineffectual medicaments may stimulate the evolution of more virulent strains.

The lowering of mortality which occurred before the present century was due less to more effective cures than to changes which either impeded the direct transfer of micro-organisms from one body to another (by greater cleanliness and the use of antiseptics) or eliminated the vectors (i.e. animal transferers such as lice or rats). The equivalent of the former for sexually-transmitted diseases is the condom, which helped to contain syphilis and gonorrhoea before the invention of penicillin. Though greatly recommended in the British government's handouts as a safe method of avoiding Aids, their reliability has been questioned by some venerologists. Nevertheless, there is little doubt that, if correctly used with an antiseptic jelly, they reduce the risk by a substantial factor: perhaps between 7 and 12. As saliva also contains the virus, perhaps the risk could be further reduced by condoms for kissing. (Ambulance personnel are already equipped with protective gadgets for mouth-to-mouth resuscitation.) However, because of the remaining margin of unreliability – as well as the consequences of negligence – it is unlikely that the use of condoms would suffice to stem the spread in conditions of great and general promiscuity.

(4) Changes in the pattern of human behaviour

An adaptation to a disease may also be achieved solely through changes in the pattern of behaviour, without recourse to any technical means, if infection is transmitted through direct bodily contacts which may be avoided by voluntary acts. This was the case in pre-modern times with leprosy which was probably prevented from spreading even more widely by the isolation of lepers, while the curtailment of promiscuity by Puritanism helped to contain syphilis. Having total power over their animals, farmers are able to stop the spread of infectious disease in their herds solely by preventing contacts between the infected and uninfected animals, totally isolating or killing the former.

On the assumption that Aids remains incurable and continues to be transmitted almost solely by sexual contacts (apart from sharing needles and careless blood transfusions), and given that condoms do not give foolproof protection, its spread can be contained only by reducing sexual contacts between the infected and uninfected. A complete stoppage of the spread could be achieved only by reducing such contacts to zero. These contacts could be prevented or reduced by the following methods:

(1) *Killing the carriers*, as is done by farmers with their herds.

(2) *Total isolation of the carriers*, as is also done by farmers and was the case with lepers.

(3) *A general reduction in the number of partners*, tending towards absolute monogamy, which entails premarital chastity and absolute fidelity within marriage. Even if the latter pattern became universal, it would not prevent all new infections through sexual relations because some people might marry carriers who have been infected through an accident. Nevertheless, the nearer a population could approach the condition of universal and absolute monogamy, the slower would be the spread of the disease, as long as non-sexual infections remained an unimportant source. This is because an accidental carrier could infect only his or her spouse and their children, who would not normally live long enough to infect others through sexual acts. However, although there are individuals and small groups who have adhered to absolute monogamy, and there are societies where this pattern is or was common, there is no record of a large society where it was universal or even nearly universal. So, we cannot expect an extirpation of Aids – or even an arrest of its spread – from such a reaction, although a very substantial reduction of the rate of spread could be achieved if a strong trend in this direction set in, even if it resulted in a curtailment of promiscuity rather than a universalisation of absolute monogamy.

(4) *Voluntary abstention on the part of the carriers* from intercourse with partners not known to be infected. For this to have any effect two conditions must be fulfilled:
   (a) All the carriers must know that they are infected and must be able to find out who else is infected.
   (b) They must be altruistic enough to forgo or limit their pleasure for the sake of other people's health.
The first of these conditions would require widespread, periodic and reliable testing, in view of the long latency of the disease which can be dormant for seven or perhaps even fourteen years, as otherwise the healthy carriers could not know that they are infected. If testing were to be voluntary, it would also depend entirely on altruism, because it amounts to a self-sacrifice to want

to spoil one's pleasures and one's peace of mind by learning that one has an incurable disease which will soon bring a painful death. From a purely selfish viewpoint, someone may have an incentive to ask for a test only if the danger which they have incurred was so small that they feel confident that the test will dispel their anxiety. So both the aforementioned conditions depend on altruism.

To expect so much altruism is even more unrealistic than to imagine that all 'public servants' are motivated solely by concern for the general welfare without regard for their own interests, particularly as among the carriers of Aids there is likely to be a disproportionate number of alienated individuals, because the risk increases with the preference for promiscuity which is connected with cold self-centred sensuality or loveless vanity. So people who are most likely to catch Aids are also least likely to be motivated by concern for others. To realise how silly it is to imagine Aids could be stopped by appeals to altruism, it is enough to think about the vast number of people who behave in a thoroughly anti-social manner: they are cruel to children, ill-treat and exploit their partners, elicit love by lies and then enjoy the grief of the jilted lover, abandon their children and so on. Equally silly is the naive faith in counselling, the only solid effect of which is to provide employment for social workers. There might be some point in trying to persuade people to take precautions by stimulating their fear of the disease, although even here the effect is doubtful. Innumerable people have been advised again and again not to smoke, drive dangerously or overeat, but they still go on. Nevertheless, some have stopped, albeit more often out of fear for themselves than a wish not to endanger others. In any case, everyday observation as well as psychological research teach us that conscience and altruism are formed early in life. So those who have reached sexual maturity without developing them, will not suddenly acquire these dispositions just because a social worker talks to them. Even from the viewpoint of a carrier's own welfare, counselling is pretty futile. Believers might be helped by a priest, who can unburden them of guilt and cheer them by an assurance of happiness after death. Thus, an irreligious sufferer might gain some relief through a conversion. In contrast, an irreligious social worker can say nothing to make death and suffering less sorrowful. True, people often feel better when they can talk to someone about their troubles, but for this purpose it is best to have someone who is in the same boat. Moreover, why should there be special solicitude for the victims of Aids? Dying from any painful illness is equally bad. Why not counsel everybody who has a terminal illness . . . or even every old person who must die soon? The fuss about counselling can be explained in the first place by the common human hankering after magic cures; secondly by the expansionist tendency of the social work bureaucracy; and thirdly by the influence of the homosexual lobby. In Minneapolis, homosexuals are specially recruited as social workers.

We can conclude that no hope can be placed in any method of containing Aids which must rely on altruism among the carriers. There is no doubt that fear among the uninfected is a far stronger and more reliable motive. Undoubtedly there will always be a few carriers who will be guided (or at least influenced) by a concern for others, but there will be enough of the irresponsible kind to ensure a continued spread of the disease, if this matter were to depend on their attitude alone. Furthermore, the good effects of the restraint on the part of the conscientious will be outweighed by the behaviour of the malicious who deliberately want to infect others – often as many as possible – out of the desire for diffuse vengeance. This sentiment was expressed by a male prostitute interviewed in London who said: 'they have fucked me to death, so I'll fuck them to death.'

(5) The introduction of the custom of medico-sexual segregation

As during the long stage of latency the carriers neither show nor feel any symptoms, any method of preventing intercourse between the infected and uninfected requires three conditions to be fulfilled:

(a) A prior detection through diagnostic tests.
(b) A method of demarcating the two categories which would permit mutual recognition.
(c) Some kind of a barrier to intercourse between categories.

(a) The present tests – which detect antibodies but not the virus – form an insufficient basis for sorting individuals because of the time lag of about seven months between the start of the infection and its detectability, during which the carrier is (or at least may be) infectious. But apparently a better test is in the offing which will detect the virus directly. Nevertheless, so long as the disease remains incurable, even a perfect test can achieve nothing unless it leads to steps which prevent intercourse between the infected and the uninfected. But the first step must be to make sure that all the carriers are identified.

It must be noted that random testing would permit an assessment of general trends but could provide no basis for preventive action. Even more futile would be anonymous testing which would leave even the tested carriers unidentified. Tests, the results of which would be communicated only to the testees, would be only a shade less futile as a preventive step because only altruistic or conscientious men and women would forfeit pleasures which endanger only others and incur other trouble, by revealing the dreadful secret to actual or potential partners. Given that altruism is scarce while there are many thoroughly irresponsible or even antisocial people, not to speak of outright sadists, general testing could reduce infections only if people were somehow compelled to reveal results, or have them revealed by someone else.

(b)   As most patterns of segregation which have existed so far were or are orientated towards excluding people from privileges, the social barriers restricted connubiality, commensality and conviviality rather than sheer physical contact. The exception was the Hindu custom of untouchability, which may have evolved, at least partly, under the influence of the fear of disease. Consequently they needed marks which permitted instant recognition – such as different dress, manners, way of speaking or deportment.

If Aids could be transmitted by breath or a slight touch, segregation for medical reasons would also require marks recognisable at a distance. As things appear to stand now, contagion takes place only through an intimate contact – either sexual or medical – with the body fluids. So, there is no need for marks recognisable at sight. In principle cards would do but they would be impractical in medical emergencies as well as in sexual advances. It might be better if people wore bracelets or necklaces (like soldiers' identification numbers) where the date and result of testing, as well as the particulars needed for identification, could be imprinted in a form difficult to counterfeit. So people would not be marked on the street but their condition would easily be ascertained when a closer physical contact was initiated or envisaged.

Marking could be either obligatory or voluntary, although there would be little point in having obligatory testing without the obligation to have a certificate in some form and to be ready to show it when demanded. If the testing and marking were done by a private institution, the credibility of the certificates would depend on the reputation of the issuer. Testing and carrying badges or certificates might be voluntary in law but obligatory in fact if anyone not possessing a badge of health would automatically be treated as infected.

In his forthcoming book about this problem (which I had the privilege of reading in typescript) Christopher Monckton proposes that testing ought to be obligatory for everyone between sixteen and sixty-five, and repeated at least once a year. Individual results would be revealed to the testees who, if not found to be infected, would have the right to obtain a certificate to this effect, which would be of such a kind that it could be displayed. To prevent fraud, it would have the photograph, personal data and the date of the test. Monckton insists that there ought to be no obligation to have or display these certificates but this seems to me to be a mere placation of liberal susceptibilities because nothing could be achieved by obligatory testing without obligatory segregation. No law would be needed if the uninfected came to regard the certificates as an indispensable condition of sex-worthiness, while anyone who did not have one would automatically be treated as untouchable. Otherwise the only result of compulsory testing would be the knowledge (as distinct from the present guessing) of how the infection is spreading . . . which would be valuable but would not amount to prevention.

Monckton takes into account the delay between infection and the appearance of antibodies in the test (usually three to seven months) and he admits that the procedure would not prevent contagion by the recently infected. Nevertheless, he argues (on the basis of calculation and computer modelling) that the probability of infection would be greatly reduced, particularly among people who do not change partners very often, and the spread of the disease would be much slower. This could be an important achievement, particularly if a cure were to be discovered in the meantime.

My reservation about Monckton's proposal is that it is not evident that obligatory testing would help much if the preventive measure of excluding the infected from sexual relations with the

uninfected either did not materialise or resulted from social pressure rather than a law. So, why not also leave the enforcement of
testing to social pressure? Perhaps a social convention might
emerge which will require the display of a sex-worthiness
certificate on pain of being treated as untouchable without it.
There is plenty of scope here for voluntary organisations and
propaganda. The only advantage of obligatory tests would be
that nobody would have the excuse that he or she could not
afford it, did not have the time or forgot about it.

(c) In a well-ordered polity it would be possible to enforce an
obligation of general testing, although, without support from
public opinion, there might be enough evasion to make the law
largely ineffective. It would be much more difficult – indeed
impossible – to prevent by law intercourse between the infected
and uninfected, because it is beyond the power even of a
totalitarian state to stamp out illicit copulation. There are many
historical examples – ranging from the attempts by the Roman
emperor Diocletian to control prices to 'the Prohibition' in the
USA in the thirties – of laws which remained a dead letter largely
because they were broken by the agents entrusted with their
enforcement. Bribery, nepotism, favouritism and collusion are
common features of bureaucratic machines. If a government
were to take upon itself the task of stopping Aids without
backing from a fairly unanimous public opinion, it would find it
easier to kill or intern the carriers than to oversee everybody's
sexual activities. Even such drastic methods, moreover, would
be ineffective unless accompanied by a policy of seclusion,
similar to that of Tokugawa Japan, with a prohibition of foreign
travel, severe limitations on entry, strict supervision of visitors
as well as the testing of all arrivals, followed by an expulsion of
all infected foreigners and the isolation or killing of infected
returners. Such procedures could not be adopted by a polity
dependent on foreign trade or where there is much movement
across the frontiers.

Methods of prevention compared

If the carriers are neither killed nor interned and continue to move
about freely, then their sexual access to the uninfected can be
impeded only by one of the three other methods listed earlier, of
which voluntary restraint on their part must be discounted as of

little practical importance. So, there are in fact only two non-statist behavioural methods of prevention: one is universal absolute monogamy, and the other the practice of untouchability or medico-sexual segregation. There is a considerable difference between them in respect of likely prevalence. As we know of no society where absolute monogamy was followed by everybody, we can assume that the trend away from promiscuity, inspired by the fear of Aids, will stop well short of this ideal type. On the other hand, the custom of untouchability has been followed very thoroughly during centuries in a number of societies – most notably in India. True, the Indian caste system was and is sanctioned by the religion – which would not be the case with medico-sexual segregation. The latter, however, would be prompted by objectively founded fear. Apart from the foregoing empirical pointer, an inferential argument can also be adduced why medico-sexual segregation is more likely to become prevalent than absolute monogamy: it is that one needs much more unflagging self-control to follow absolute monogamy – particularly when through bad luck or the lack of foresight one has landed up with an incompatible partner – than to avoid a certain category of people . . . especially if the latter constitute only a minority.

Sexual contacts are easier to prevent if there is a ban on conviviality and commensality with the forbidden class or classes – this was the common practice in many societies, including the British colonies until the end of the Empire, and it is still practised in South Africa and India, as well as in Japan towards the Eta caste. Though often in a more blurred form, such practices are common throughout the world. In consequence of the tendency of attitudes to spread, it is likely that medico-sexual segregation will be accompanied by a more generalised segregation, which could also be fostered by the fear of non-sexual contagion, which is unlikely but not proven to be impossible.

Given that perfect thoroughness is unlikely to be achieved in the practice of either method, a combination of both is likely to be needed to achieve an adequate degree of prevention. There is between them a relationship of mutual compensation: that is, if one of them is implemented to a lesser extent, then the other must be employed more if a given degree of prevention of contacts is to be attained. Thus, those who do not like the idea of untouchability ought to advocate universal absolute monogamy and vice versa. True, this compensatory relationship between the two methods is complicated by the factor of 'condomisation' – i.e. how prevalent is the use of condoms? But in view of the insufficient reliability of this technical method of avoiding infection, the need for the behavioural methods remains . . . and so does the need to choose between various doses thereof.

From the viewpoint of the interests of the uninfected, the constraints of absolute monogamy would be more irksome than the creation of a class of untouchables, because the latter adaptation would leave the uninfected some freedom – such as trying out a partner before committing oneself for good or escaping from an unhappy marriage – even though this would be very far from the promiscuity of the permissive era.

So long as the infected constitute a small minority, they can easily be cast into an untouchable class. If they become a majority, the segregation would have to be much more rigorous to enable the uninfected minority to survive.

Segregation of the infected has two inherent weaknesses which would remain even if it were unremittingly and unanimously pursued with the aid of tests capable of showing the infection immediately after its occurrence. One of these weaknesses stems from the possibility of cheating, as people do with credit cards. This could be largely obviated by technical improvements, which would make it more difficult to counterfeit or to use stolen discs or cards. Such improvements might be impeded by prejudices like those which prevent the British banks from curtailing fraud with credit cards by including photos, fingerprints or personal data and descriptions. Less remediable is the second weakness: the inevitable interval between tests. Clearly it is impossible to test people every hour, every day or every week. Yet, it is perfectly possible for an individual to become infected immediately after the test and to infect others before the next test. For this reason it would be impossible to make promiscuity safe simply by confining it within the circle of certificate holders.

Most commonly promiscuity is practised with promiscuous partners who, even if they have certificates, might have been infected during the interval between the tests, particularly if they cannot be trusted to be prudent enough to use condoms with due care. It follows that finding a new partner even within the circle of certificate holders would have to be a longish and cautious procedure, very different from the casual picking up which became common during the permissive era.

Another and related consequence of these circumstances will be the enhanced importance of a reputation of being responsible, as well as of a knowledge of who has what kind of reputation. To insure safety from infection, medico-sexual segregation would have to exclude not only those who have failed or did not undergo a sex-worthiness test, but also those who do not inspire confidence about having behaved prudently since the last test. This entails an upwards valuation of truthfulness – a trait which is also a necessary condition of the prevalence of monogamy.

Faithfulness to one partner affords no protection unless it is reciprocal. The old-fashioned code of behaviour of the Mediterranean kind, which puts curbs only on women while giving men a dispensation, provides no barrier. The danger of lethal infection puts a great value on trustworthiness and veracity. Consequently, these virtues will be restored to their status while deceit will again be regarded as a grave transgression. This will entail a reversal of the recent trend towards flippancy in these matters, exemplified by an article in the *Guardian* where the author advised women, who fear that they might have caught a venereal disease in a casual encounter, about which is the best lie to tell their husbands as an excuse for refraining from intercourse. Another example of this attitude is the twist given to the divorce law by trendy judges who have decreed (flaunting as well as undermining the moral sentiments of the people) that no amount of adultery and deceit can affect a woman's entitlement to life-long maintenance by the ex-husband. Given the power of the legal profession to give every law a twist which enlarges the amount of litigation and augments lawyers' fees, most iniquities and absurdities of the divorce law may remain for a long time but the lighthearted view of marital deceit will no doubt be abandoned when the disease has made more substantial inroads.

Condoms, of course, reduce the chances of infection but, apart from the imperfect technical reliability, there is a behavioural risk in relying solely on them, which stems from negligence, impulsiveness or selfishness, all of which can be greatly aggravated by alcohol or drugs which reduce not only the sense of responsibility but also fear. So, condoms alone are unlikely to stop Aids. To achieve this, they must be accompanied by a trend towards monogamy and the custom of medico-sexual segregation. The latter two adaptive responses, however, would not obviate the need for condoms, unless they were practised with a degree of thoroughness which is very unlikely, otherwise some risk would still be incurred in entering into a marriage, let alone a less stable union, unless it were preceded by a test as well as a quarantine period, until tests with immediate efficacity are available. Given that a certain length of acquaintance is needed for the growth of trust, people would have to use condoms if they wanted to have a little room for trying out potential partners, even if their style of life was very far from the permissiveness of the recent times. Even with a condom, there would be some risk in trying it out with someone who did not appear to be trustworthy or whose way of life increased the probability of infection. So even with condoms and a trend away from promiscuity, the custom of medico-sexual segregation would be useful to those anxious to avoid the risk.

The use of condoms is likely to have two side effects which many will regard as good. The first is the reduction of illegitimate births. The second is the encouragement of monogamy, due to the reduction of pleasure in dangerous adulterous copulation. There might be an increased preference for unencumbered intercourse with a trustworthy spouse (even if her or his sex appeal is moderate or on the wane) in comparison with a more exciting possible partner with whom artificial safeguards would be advisable.

Consuetudinal versus socio-surgical adaptation

The examination of the way in which the various methods of preventing the spread of infection are linked, leads us to the conclusion that adaptation, which results from a spontaneous change in customs and attitudes – and which for this reason we may call consuetudinal adaptation – must consist of three elements:

(1) A trend away from promiscuity and towards monogamy.
(2) A custom of medico-sexual segregation (which requires testing and demarcation).
(3) The use of condoms in any relationship of transition or trial.

Customs and values cannot be changed as quickly as laws or decrees. So, a consuetudinal adaptation must take a long time whereas medico-social surgery – that is, physical elimination of the infected – can be quick. For this reason the latter, though brutal in its methods, may entail less suffering in the end because it permits an extirpation of the disease while still only a very few are infected, whereas a consuetudinal adaptation is unlikely to take place until the danger stares everyone in the face – that is, when the sufferers are numerous and everybody knows one. Furthermore, a socio-surgical adaptation may alter the public's way of life less than a consuetudinal one, because once the infected have been eliminated, the rest can live more or less as before, whereas the latter adaptation involves a change in behaviour patterns which must be maintained indefinitely . . . or at least until either the virus disappears or a cure is found.

Medico-social surgery can be most easily undertaken and executed by a totalitarian government, especially as it has to be followed by withdrawal from contacts with abroad. So we arrive at the paradoxical conclusion that sexual freedom might best be vouchsafed by totalitarianism.

ASPECTS OF CONSUETUDINAL ADAPTATION

Owing to the slowness of consuetudinal adaptation, many people must die before it can take place. So,one of the side effects is likely to be the decline (or even disappearance) of unemployment, particularly as Aids strikes mostly young adults.

Barring medico-social surgery, no government can do anything decisive to prevent the spread of Aids. All it can do is to try to persuade people to change their ways. If infection quickly produced incapacity or clearly visible symptoms, there would be no need for campaigns to scare people off the invisible danger. And how effective will they be?

My guess is that they will retard somewhat the spread of infection but not arrest it, because appeals to prudence have little, if any, effect on large sectors of the population. At the moment condomless heterosexual promiscuity is (outside Africa) less dangerous than smoking. Yet plently of people smoke. True, fewer people smoke now than ten years ago but the reduction occurred mainly among educated people. Smoking remains prevalent among the least educated and least intelligent sections of the population. But more significant, as an indication of human proneness to disregard remote dangers, is the fact that there are still many smokers among very intelligent and highly educated people (including scientists and doctors) fully acquainted with statistical reasoning and evidence, and who are conscientious and considerate in other respects, but are nevertheless unable to overcome the craving which endangers their own and their family's health. Even among Greens – ostensibly devoted to keeping the air pure – there are smokers who discredit their pleading. The sexual impulse in the young and healthy is more universal and not easier to control than the craving for tobacco. Innumerable people have risked shame, torture or fatal disease under its promptings. Even ferocious tyrants (Henry VIII for example) have been cuckolded.

There are drugs much more dangerous than tobacco, in their physiological effects as well as because of their illegality, which find an increasing number of devotees. More common than an addiction to lethal drugs, though less common than smoking, is dangerous driving. Is it likely that people who are ready to risk their life or health for the sake of such indulgence will be willing to reduce their pleasure by using condoms, let alone practise premarital chastity, particularly as an unseen danger makes no impact on people without imagination? The fear of Aids will acquire a greater motivating force when nearly everybody has seen somebody suffering and dying, but even then there will be many people who will disregard the danger. If their number approaches that of smokers, the spread of Aids will be very rapid, but it is likely to slow down when most imprudent or ignorant people have been infected, so that a further increase in the number of the infected would have to occur through accidents, the most common of which would be burst condoms.

Although they are likely to be picked on because they are conspicuous, I doubt whether prostitutes will be the chief spreaders of the disease in the more developed countries because (apart from those who are on drugs) they are professionals who go about their jobs coolly. Infection is more likely to occur among excited young lovers who may have forgotten or lost their condoms or cannot resist the temptation of a more intense pleasure. The least likely to escape infection are promiscuous drunkards and drug addicts, even apart from the question of contaminated needles. Another factor is superstitions which prompt reliance on amulets and incantations. This is very important in Africa where most people believe in witchcraft, but far from unimportant even in the most highly industrialised countries.

In developed countries (with the exception of those willing to resort to medico-social surgery) the earliest general calamity caused by Aids will be the breakdown of the health services. Provision of medical care for every sick person depends on there being enough healthy individuals who can be spared from other kinds of necessary work – which is utterly impossible if the sick outnumber the healthy, and becomes practically impossible long before this ratio is reached. This factor operates with particular force in the case of Aids, which strikes mainly at young adults, in contrast to most other epidemics which attack more virulently and frequently the old and children. According to a recent estimate in Britain the cost of caring for a sufferer is about £20,000, and by 1997 all existing hospital beds will be needed for Aids patients if the present trend continues. If this were to happen, then either the numbers of hospitals and medical personnel would have to be doubled or other illnesses would be left untreated. Even if the provision of medical services were to be doubled, it would be overwhelmed a couple of years later. Such calculations have prompted the government to jettison deeply-rooted notions of propriety in the publicity campaign to induce people to use condoms.

The swamping of hospitals and surgeries will force the policy makers and the medical profession to face squarely the issue which up till now they have preferred to dodge: the necessity of abandoning the hopeless cases in order to be able to help those who may recover. This is the choice which battlefield surgeons were often compelled to make – a practice known under its French name 'triage'.

Even without Aids the medical services cannot keep up with the need. In party political exchanges, the opposition usually blames this on the stinginess of the party in power – which may be justified in some respects. There is, unfortunately, a deeper cause: the inherently self-defeating nature of medical progress. As more ailments and disabilities become treatable, the work load increases, particularly as very often the cure is not definitive and treatment must be repeated. More often than not a patient whose death has been prevented adds to the demand for future services. The practice of prolonging life regardless of its quality – even when it is nothing but constant pain without hope – makes it debatable whether medical progress has really improved the balance between happiness and suffering. What is not debatable is that this practice has stretched medical resources to the point where they do not suffice for a proper treatment of curable diseases. Nevertheless, in our euphemistic civilisation this issue is strenuously avoided. An even stronger taboo surrounds the other self-defeating mechanism inherent in medical progress: the increase in deleterious genes in the population as their carriers are enabled with the help of medicaments and operations not only to survive but also to procreate. No discussion of this grave problem is allowed by the consensual censorship because it would puncture the pipe dream that our species can permanently escape from selection for reproduction which operates throughout nature. The temporary suspension of this selection, which has occurred during recent decades in the affluent societies has been unceasingly augmenting the need for medical services despite the elimination of epidemics.

The flood of sufferers from Aids will put an end to the aspiration that everyone ought to be able to obtain medical treatment to the limit of technological possibilities. Many people will have to be abandoned – if not helped to die – and the only choice will be between *triage* – that is rationing on the basis of estimates of likely benefits from treatment – and allocation through the market, in which case wealthy incurables will receive most attention while the poor will be dying of easily curable ailments. Such a situation might prompt a conflict of an unprecedented type: a kind of class struggle of the curable poor against the incurable rich for scarce medical resources, which might be justified by an ideology somewhat analogous to national socialism where socialist solidarity was restricted to a certain group and directed against another. The enemy would be the wealthy sufferers from Aids who were taking up all the available medical resources.

Sufferers from Aids will no doubt be debarred from access to medical services as soon as their number grows to the point where they become a serious burden. This outcome will also be promoted by the self-interest of the medical personnel, increasingly unwilling to risk infection, particularly when the effort can bear no fruit. So long as the sufferers are few, it is possible to find enough altruistic nurses to care for them. But the supply of such people is limited, and there might be a flight from this profession if an attempt is made to coerce them to do what they don't want to. The only tenable way of alleviating the sufferers' fate would be to set up hospices staffed by people who are infected but not yet disabled. However, merely providing them with shelter, food, heating and clothing might become a heavy burden on the rest of the population. Any drug which merely prolongs the illness will add to the burden. As mentioned earlier, the depletion of the labour force ought to bring mass unemployment to an end, particularly as the incidence of infection seems to be especially high in the class of unemployables.

Aids has radically changed the significance of imprisonment.

Given that buggery is rife in jails, even a short stay there may in fact amount to a death sentence, particularly for a man who is young and nice-looking but not very strong. Idleness and overcrowding multiply temptations and opportunities, while making it difficult to resist importuning, intimidation or rape. Prisons are perhaps the most important channels for spreading infection among heterosexuals because most inmates practise homosexuality only as a substitute and find women as soon as they are released. These facts will call into question the current dogma that imprisonment is the only acceptable form of punishment apart from fines. Stocks, the pillory, even lashes are a milder punishment than being put into a situation where one is almost certain to catch Aids.

Aids has made rape a much graver offence. This applies also to the homosexual rape of a man, which hitherto was regarded as a less tragic event because it cannot lead to a pregnancy. Owing to the increased danger, seduction of the young will be more severely punished.

The arrival of Aids has defeated the efforts of homosexuals to make themselves acceptable. The word 'gay' has become a cruel joke, as being liable to catch Aids – let alone having it – is hardly a reason for gaiety. Even before the disease appeared, most parents did not want their sons to be homosexual. Now they have an additional and very strong motive for trying to prevent it. They might try to achieve this through a much stricter supervision of boys' activities, avoidance of boarding schools, and a purge of homosexuals from the teaching profession and other positions entailing contact with the young, such as sports organisers.

To the heterosexual majority, pure homosexuals have become a burden (because of their disproportionate claims on medical resources) and a nuisance, to be avoided because of the uncertainty about non-sexual transmission of the disease through a contact with bodily fluids. But they do not constitute a direct danger. In contrast, bisexuals do bring the disease from the more heavily infected circle to the majority, who therefore have a good reason for turning against them. The outcome might be a custom of strict delimitation similar to that which was practiced by some American Indian tribes, where homosexuals (though perfectly tolerated) had to wear a distinct dress, live in a separate part of the village and were severely punished for any sexual approaches to women.

The collapse of the welfare state and the unavoidable abandonment of the mass of sufferers to their fate will foster a change of

outlook and values in the direction of ideologies which justify
individual and group selfishness, as the Puritan notion of predestination justified the withholding of alms. The egalitarianism which
has dominated public opinion since the Second World War (and
intermittently since the First) may be displaced by doctrines
somewhat reminiscent of the Nazi view that defective individuals
and groups ought to be eliminated in the interests of the health
and strength of the bulk of the nation. Another route away from
egalitarianism leads through (what some people call) Thatcherism –
that is, a return to a capitalism inspired by the Victorian attitude
to the less fortunate, epitomised in the saying 'let the devil take
the hindmost', and purged of the redistributive policies and social
security introduced around the two World Wars in response to the
need to mobilise the masses and inspire them with patriotic ardour.
The established parties may hesitate to take steps which might
allay the public's fear but which would also entail the casting of
many of the top people into the class of untouchables. This might
give a chance to the aspiring politicians on the margins of society
to set up new parties devoted to ruthless programs. The ground
would be prepared by the collapse of the ideal of the caring society,
which would open the gate for venting other resentments such as
the dislike of immigrants (especially of a different race) and their
descendants.

The presence of the victims of Aids in state schools and hospitals –
which the healthy will regard as a dangerous infestation – will give
a great boost to private schools and hospitals, where a thorough
segregation can be practised without governmental intervention,
or even despite laws to the contrary. People may be prepared to
work alongside a carrier, but be reluctant to expose to such contacts
their children, who are much more likely to be involved in
accidents, fights or other acts which lead to contact with blood or
bodily effluents.

Given that contagion can be avoided by a personal decision (or
rather a joint decision of two individuals) the victims will be to a
large extent self-selected in consequence of individual and group
characteristics, such as lack of foresight or self-control, ignorance
(which may be due to low intelligence), the strength and wayward-
ness of their sexual desire, the inability to form enduring relationships or a predilection for alcohol and drugs. Now, the will and
the ability to control sexual desire sufficiently to choose a partner
carefully, or to take adequate precautions, tends to be connected
with the more general ability to defer gratification for the sake of

more distant goals, which is likely to reveal itself in other spheres of life as thrift and industriousness. So, by and large (and setting apart the old people dependent on state pensions or public assistance) the sexual untouchables will be more numerous among economic failures. It follows that the barrier of sexual untouchability will accentuate the chasm in the class structure which is developing for other reasons (namely, automation in combination with the ecological constraints on economic growth) along the boundary between the employed and fairly affluent skilled class and the surplus class consisting of people who are either unfit for any work, or only for unskilled work for which there is no demand.

Despite the considerable overlapping of the health and economic boundaries at the lowest end of the social ladder, there is no equivalent correspondence at the other end, because one section of the rich has been struck by Aids harder than any other class (apart perhaps from down-and-out drug addicts) namely, the practitioners of the entertainment industry. As they surpass all other professions in their inclination towards promiscuity, homo-sexuality and drugs, their ranks will be drastically depleted, and they will be replaced by newcomers of a different type.

The entertainers as well as the advertisers may also lose econom-ically, because their wealth and influence rest largely upon their art of titillating lust; and, if people are obliged to restrain it, they may wish to avoid spectacles which whet it. So, the hidden persuaders will lose their most important tool for manipulating minds.

As an aside, I shall venture a forecast about popular music. The older style – as exemplified by the songs of Bing Crosby or the tunes of George Gershwin – had a romantic and sentimental flavour (as did the traditional European folk love songs) whereas today's pop music is orgiastic. The former echoes a yearning for the object of unsatisfied desire, while the latter reflects an expectation of the immediate gratification of every passing impulse, without a trace of what Freud calls sublimation. The end of safe and uninhibited indulgence will cause many people to experience a yearning for inaccessible or awaited delights, which will make the orgiastic music unattractive and enhance the appeal of romantic and sentimental styles.

It is less clear what will be the impact of Aids on pornography because here two tendencies oppose each other. On the one hand, frustration often inspires pruriency and voyeurism, and therefore may raise the demand for pornography. On the other hand, if you

Appendix One

must keep to the straight and narrow path, you may enjoy more
peace of mind if you avoid sights and sounds which conjure up
ungratifiable appetites or dangerous temptations. Perhaps both
inclinations could be satisfied, and mental comfort maximised, if
pornography became more discreet – that is, continued to be
accessible to those who deliberately seek it, but ceased to be foisted
upon those who prefer to avoid it. In contrast, nothing good is
achieved by harassing obscure publishers and booksellers, while
condoning unsolicited titillation on television and publicly displayed
posters, which is the policy of the present government in Britain.

The ravages of Aids, as well as the burden and danger which
the infected represent for the rest, might prompt a change in the
present attitudes to suicide and euthanasia which stem from
primitive stages of civilisation. There are no rational grounds for
trying to prevent a suicide of someone whose life is sheer misery
without hope. If such a person is also a danger and burden to
others, it will be a deed of benevolence if he puts an end to his
existence. Rather than a posthumous insult (implied by the usual
imputation of unsound mind) he deserves praise and gratitude.
The same is true of voluntary euthanasia except that the fact of
assistance creates a need for safeguards to prevent concealment of
murder. The possibility of a small increase of undetected murders
must be set against the enormity of suffering caused by excessive
prolongation of life which the recent scientific advances have made
possible. Indeed, if we take into account how many more people
go through hell before they die (and for how much longer), then
we may doubt whether the balance sheet of medical progress is in
fact positive in relation to the goal of increasing the sum of
happiness and reducing suffering. This goal also justifies involun-
tary euthanasia of the very sick who are clearly suffering but are
unable to speak, as well as infanticide in cases of severe defects
which make a life of misery inevitable. It is rather absurd to
permit abortions for non-vital economic reasons while punishing
indubitable mercy killings. An adaptation to the situation created
by the recent advances in medicine and pharmacology is hindered
by mental inertia, superstitions and mankind's appetite for grati-
fying delusions. It is possible that the shock of Aids and the
obvious impossibility of perpetuating the present arrangements
might induce an adjustment.

NON-ADAPTIVE REACTIONS

So far we have discussed the consequences of (at least partly) rational reactions – that is, of actions inspired by fears for which there are some real grounds. Most of these reactions can also be regarded as adaptive because they are likely to (or, at least might) reduce the danger of infection and therefore the speed of its spread. The historical examples are, to repeat, the isolation of lepers and Puritanism. Now let us examine the possibility and likelihood of reactions which might be described as irrational (in the sense of being inspired by groundless fears) or inadaptive – that is, unlikely to arrest or even delay the spread of the disease, as was the case with the witch hunts. Such irrational or inadaptive reactions might ensue from the operation of some general tendencies of human behaviour.

The tendency to overshoot the point of adaptation

Looking at collective reactions to changing circumstances, we can see the tendency to overshoot the point of adaptation. This tendency has been well studied in economics in connection with business cycles and other fluctuations on the markets, where a scramble for shares or commodities is often followed by equally wild selling – 'bulls' turning quickly and massively into 'bears' or the other way round. The 'cobweb theorem' postulates that price adjustments normally reach the point of equilibrium through a series of diminishing overshots.

The normative tendency

Working in the same direction (once the trend sets in) is the tendency which a nineteenth century theorist of jurisprudence, Gustaf von Ihering, called 'the normative tendency of the actual' – the tendency of any pattern of behaviour (no matter how fortuitous might be its origin) to acquire a normative (or, if you prefer, a prescriptive) charge simply in consequence of its duration. In other words, if people happen to go on doing certain things in a certain way long enough, they will soon come to feel that this is how it ought to be done, and that it is improper or even wicked to do it in a different way. Without using Ihering's term, many other writers have mentioned this tendency in connection with problems of how customs, morals and manners emerge and hold sway. This tendency is so ubiquitous that it deserves a snappier label than Ihering's. I propose 'normatisation' for the process, and 'normativity' for the quality – that is the degree to which a pattern of behaviour has acquired a prescriptive force. 'Normatisation' must not be confused with 'normalisation', where the root word 'norm' is used in the sense of statistical regularity rather than an obligatory (or at least prescribed) custom. The relevance of this concept to our forecast is that if people abstain from carnal pleasures for purely pragmatic prudential reasons, the tendency to normatise will lead them eventually to feel that abstention is good while indulgence is wicked.

The tendency to make a virtue of a necessity

Closely interwoven with normatisation, which derives its strength from the sheer inertia of culture, is the tendency to make a virtue out of a necessity. The Polish Jews had a saying 'if you don't have what you like, you like what you have'. The tendency to make a virtue out of a necessity can go much further: you begin to feel that it is wrong to have what you don't have, that it is laudable not to have it, and that anyone who has it is wicked. Through this mental process, frustrations accepted out of necessity acquire the status of virtues, whose practitioners are admired while the infringers are despised and eagerly punished. This tendency plays such an important role in the emergence and crystallisation of customs and morals that it merits a name: I propose 'virtuation'. One of the factors which help its operation is envy, which is a universal human characteristic albeit subject to wide variations. These variations depend, no doubt, on many factors (including the genetic) but the most important seems to be the amount of frustration: frustrated people tend to be more envious than the contented. The relationship however, might be somewhat complicated by the inverse causation: those prone to envy are more likely to be frustrated and less contented.

The tendency to virtuate – to make a virtue out of necessity – provided the link between the epidemic of syphilis and the puritanical abhorrence of all pleasures of the flesh rather than a mere abstention from their more dangerous kinds. Given that there is little evidence that human nature has changed fundamentally, it is reasonable to suppose that this tendency will prompt a somewhat similar reaction to Aids when (or if) it becomes a menace to the majority. Owing to the influence of science, however, the new version of Puritanism may be less dependent on theology.

The tendency to seek a scapegoat

The fourth tendency likely to prompt reactions going beyond the point of adaptation to danger is the inclination to find someone to blame, and preferably to punish, regardless of their real role in producing the calamity: in other words, to look for a scapegoat. We already have the verb 'to scapegoatise someone' (albeit it is used only in restricted circles in touch with psychoanalysis) which means casting him or her into the role of scapegoat. I suggest that we call 'scapegoating' the entire process of reacting to calamity by putting the blame on an individual or a minority who did not in fact cause it.

How reactions can go too far

There are several directions in which the reactions to the disease can be pushed beyond the point of adaptation by the tendencies outlined above:

Devotionalism: up to a point the growth of a religious sentiment which supports the avoidance of promiscuity may be regarded as adaptive, because it might restrain from indulgence individuals who are not cautious enough, as Puritanism probably did in the seventeenth century. However, Puritanism, as you remember, went far beyond the point of prophylaxis in its abhorrence of pleasures which could endanger nobody, such as warm water for baths, as well as in putting a taboo on speaking about sexual matters or parts. Perhaps the gratification obtained by imagining the torments of envied sinners in hell might be less strong than among celibate clerics, because the sinners would be punished in this world by Aids. The Puritan's favourite saying 'the wages of sin is death' will be even more justified than during the epidemic of syphilis. If you have to bear frustrations, you will feel more comfortable if you believe that you are achieving a greater goal than the mere preservation of good health, and that you will be rewarded for it in the afterlife. Furthermore, among the less intelligent and more ignorant part of the population the decline of religion has perhaps been less due to the influence of science and rationalism than to the desire to be free from constraints on the search for carnal pleasures, in a situation when the practical deterrents have been removed by penicillin and the pill. People who put no great value on reason and logic are inclined to adopt any belief which satisfies their cravings. What is perhaps even more important, most people revere science not because they value pure knowledge but because it brings them material goods and cures for ill-health. So, the advent of a disease against which science is helpless is likely to undermine respect for science among the masses.

A surge of religious fanaticism may help to arrest the spread of Aids by erecting taboos with a greater motivating force than mere prudence. On the other hand, however, it might bring dangers even greater than Aids. A trust that God will provide, and therefore there is no need to worry about distant dangers, might encourage the disregard of environmental dangers such as overpopulation, soil erosion, depletion of the ozone layer and pollution. Furthermore, the belief that the victory of the Faith is more important than the survival of the species, let alone of any part thereof, may make people less averse to starting nuclear war. Given the suicidal nature of such a war, no sane person can embark upon it in pursuit of an earthly goal. Not so a religious fanatic, who may welcome his own death or a holocaust as the road to heavenly bliss, as can be seen from the example of the sect who committed joint suicide in the jungle of Guatemala a few years ago, or the behaviour of Khomeini's young soldiers. That there are people who look forward to a nuclear war as the way to redeem mankind can be seen from the following passage by an American fundamentalist, Lance Lambert in *Battle for Israel* (Tyndale House Publishers, Wheaton, Illinois, 1975):

If there were a collision between the United States and Russia over Israel, China could take the opportunity of attacking Russia in the back. Thus we could have half the world locked in conflict within a matter of days. Within weeks Europe could be occupied and freed, Russia devastated, and China laid waste and the political systems centred in them destroyed. Very much of what we now call civilization would then be in ruins. Out of such catastrophe could come a period of unparalleled gospel opportunity. It would be opportunity unprecedented in the last 2,000 years, because the world would be in pieces and there would be a moral vacuum. The church of God could have possibilities for preaching and teaching such as she has never known.

The current of devotionalism may assume two forms:

(a)   A fundamentalist revival of an old religion, as is happening to some extent in the United States, and happened in a big way in Europe during the Reformation. At present the greatest revival of religious militancy can be seen in the lands of Islam, where it has been engendered not by a new disease but by the impoverishment and desperation caused mainly by overpopulation. Islamic revivalism, however, constitutes a lesser obstacle to infection than the Christian because it puts curbs on women only, while men are allowed to be randy so long as they do not interfere with other men's wives.

(b)   A rise of new religions with a puritanical streak, of which 'the Moonies' might be an example. They have the advantage of offering the comforts of the security and solidarity of a commune, as well as authoritarian and puritan strict moral guidance, supported by tenets which are so esoteric and elusive that they do not stand in clear contradiction to science, in contrast to the fundamentalist interpretations of the Bible or the Koran. Their practice of arranged marriages, usually followed by an obligation to wait several months or even years for a consummation, is well-suited to testing for Aids and a quarantine, while their recommendation of premarital chastity and the insistence on absolute marital fidelity are as if designed to eliminate the danger of infection. The more rampant the disease in the population as a whole, the more attractive will be a religion which vouchsafes an uninfected spouse, particularly when its appeal is enhanced by the prosperity created by the cult of work.

Prudential abstention may evoke a non-religious cult of asceticism which from sexual matters might spill over into a kind of spartanism. However, in the past such an outlook was invariably connected with training for war, which in the future will require even less bodily prowess than today, let alone in the past. For this reason such a reaction seems much less likely than the preceding.

Fear may prompt the craving for scapegoats which in turn may lead to forms of victimisation unrelated to the prevention of contagion, or against groups who constitute no danger – with results which are the opposite of an adaptation.

The following categories are likely to be scapegoatised:

(a)   Sexual deviants: even fully adult homosexuals, who live as
faithful couples and endanger no one thereby, may be per-
secuted; as may also be lesbians, albeit they are less likely to
transmit Aids than the heterosexuals. As it is the bisexuals who
represent a real danger to the majority, it would be a rational
policy to try to eliminate this category by enforcing a clear
demarcation and segregation in accordance with sexual orientation. However, such a rational solution might be discarded
amidst undiscriminating execration in favour of wholesale persecution of homosexuals, who then would take care to conceal
their activities, which would make the detection of bisexuals
more difficult.

(b)   Generalised xenophobia: there is a rational element in
avoiding or excluding foreigners who come from much more
infected parts of the world, although this could with equal logic
be applied to movements between towns or regions within the
same country. This concern, however, might lead to a xenophobia of which we have already seen some rather absurd examples.

Earlier in this book I have mentioned how Jews (and, more rarely,
Gipsies) have been blamed for the outbreaks of pestilence, and
how the mechanism of scapegoating provided a link between the
epidemic of syphilis and the witch hunts. Nevertheless, I doubt
whether anything very similar will occur in response to Aids,
because of our much greater understanding of natural causation,
albeit I would not go so far as to say that this is absolutely
impossible. Known or likely carriers (such as homosexuals and
drug addicts) might be treated as untouchable, but such an
avoidance would be more similar to the segregation of lepers than
to the witch hunts because the danger would not be imaginary
even if it were exaggerated. Moreover, a medico-social segregation
would decelerate the spread of the disease outside the high-risk
categories. To repeat, however, so long as there is little risk of
catching Aids outside sexual contacts, heterosexuals have little
reason to fear pure homosexuals, as the only real danger comes
from bisexuals. Nevertheless, there are two reasons why segregation of homosexuals would be less irrational than burning witches
The first is the difficulty of distinguishing pure homosexuals from
bisexuals. The second is the uncertainty about the danger from
non-sexual contacts, which is said to be very small though no

non-existent. Particularly in view of the complacency (if not mendacity) of the authorities in most countries (including Britain) about ecological dangers, many people mistrust the official assurances and prefer to err on the side of safety.

Perhaps more akin to witch hunts in respect of inadaptativeness or irrationality are some of the outbursts of xenophobia which have taken place. Segregation and screening of foreigners may serve a useful purpose where Aids has made few inroads and visitors are few (as in the case of China). In contrast, the proposals in Bavaria to test compulsorily immigrant workers (but not tourists or business travellers, nor immigrants from other regions of Germany) can be regarded as a pure placebo. Even more irrational was a similar proposal in New York, which is one of the two capitals of Aids outside Africa. On the other hand, discrimination against entrants from more heavily infected areas would be nearer to a rational precaution than to scapegoating.

DIFFERENCES BETWEEN CULTURES AND POLITIES

Their ability to extirpate Aids might give an unexpected advantage to the most seclusionist of the totalitarian systems. Thus it is quite likely that China will remain free of Aids. It has already subjected to the test the few African students which it harbours, and expelled those infected. Foreign visitors are closely watched and usually debarred from sexual contacts with the natives. The not numerous returners from abroad are put through tests and sometimes quarantines. As the carriers must still be few, they could easily be isolated in remote camps or be killed to make sure that the healthy are safe. Not only the rulers but also the ordinary Chinese have a record of ruthless social surgery. Immediately after the Revolution, the Communists extirpated the rampant addiction to opium by rounding and shooting or sending to death camps the addicts as well as the pedlars. Apart from victims of accidents, there appear to be no handicapped people in China because defective children are killed at birth. Mental defectives also seem to disappear, perhaps as a side effect of the policy of compulsory limitation of offspring.

In view of this rational ruthlessness, it would be surprising if the Chinese shrunk from exterminating (or at least totally isolating) the carriers of the Aids infection to insure the health of the rest. The non-religious puritanism, which the Chinese rulers are inculcating into the population, will in any case make the spread of Aids slower than in the more permissive societies. There is much less puritanism in the USSR which also has more contacts with the rest of the world. As its post-Stalinist élite is more influenced by Western ideas, they may be hesitant about carrying out medico-social surgery which would probably have to be on a more massive scale than in the case of China because the number of the infected might well be larger. These factors operate with an even greater force in the satellite countries of Eastern Europe. No effective preventive measures are likely to be taken in the liberal states until the catastrophe arrives in full force. The exception might be Japan, which has a liberal democratic constitution but also has networks of informal control which maintain discipline and the hierarchic sentiment. With their stronger national solidarity and exclusiveness, as well as greater individual self-control, the Japanese might be able to contain the epidemic by taking precautions, tightening the code of sexual behaviour and excluding infected visitors. They have no immigration and do not need the money from tourism. A law has already been passed which instructs customs officials to refuse entry to anyone whom they suspect of being a carrier. The unromantic attitude to marriage (still mostly occurring by arrangement between families) fits well with the need for test certificates. There would probably be very little, if any, resistance to compulsory testing of everyone.

None of these circumstances can be found in Western Europe or North America where liberalism has been transformed into an undiscriminating and pusillanimous tolerance of even the most antisocial behaviour. The politicians, moreover, have encouraged people's natural inclination to think only about immediate gratifications, regardless of long-term collective interests. To this must be added the general aversion to facing unpleasant truths, evidenced by (among many other things) the luxuriant proliferation of euphemisms. No justification for hope can be derived from the governments' records on environmental issues: while making a great fuss about peripheral issues like seat belts or corporal punishment in schools, the politicians are perfectly willing to condemn millions of people to an untimely death from cancer and other diseases caused by pollution, for the sake of not reducing the short-term profitability of certain branches of industry. Unfortunately, the masses, cretinised by the media, are also indifferent to their own long-term interests, let alone those of future generations. For example, a recent opinion poll in Britain has shown that the majority of motorists do not wish to pay more for fuel without lead, although they are ready to spend much larger sums for gimmicky gadgets.[3] Like the smokers, many of them disbelieve or disregard the scientific evidence. So, it is unlikely that anything will be done about Aids until the danger becomes so great that it stares everyone in the face. Then there will be panic but the number of the infected will be so great that it will be very difficult to do anything.

It seems that most governments are hoping that the situation will be saved by pharmacology, albeit even if a cure is invented tomorrow, there would be the formidable task of treating the large number of infected people. If the gamble fails and no cure is found, the ensuing panic is likely to put an end to liberalism, because medico-social surgery (that is, the total isolation or killing of individuals regarded as constituting a danger but not guilty of a crime) is incompatible with the idea of human rights. Nevertheless, democracy – in the sense of government by consent of the majority – could survive so long as the uninfected remained in the majority and were willing to sacrifice the rights of the minority for the sake of their own safety. However, the machinery of coercion needed for massive social surgery would most likely acquire such a momentum that a *de facto* despotism would emerge, which might resemble Nazi despotism but with the crucial difference that it would lack its militaristic and imperialistic propensities, owing to the rapid decline of the population. In a way it would be more realistic than the pseudo-racism of Hitler whose 'defence' of the purity of the race was chimerical, as there was no pure German race to be preserved. In contrast, the elimination of the carriers of Aids would amount to a real 'purification' of the population. If the numbers involved were very large, it might be impossible to maintain safeguards against the machinery of social surgery being used for unenvisaged purposes such as eliminating political opponents.

One may agree with the critics who blame the authorities for playing down the danger and for being more concerned with the comfort of the infected few than the safety of the majority. It may be that this attitude reflects the influence of the homosexual lobby. According to a writer in a magazine for homosexuals, there are about a hundred homosexuals (including bisexuals and lesbians)

in the British Parliament. Be that as it may, however, it is not easy
to visualise what the authorities could do (apart from campaigns
of persuasion) to safeguard public health without resorting to social
surgery which no one has so far advocated in public. In any case,
social surgery would require an insulation from the outside world
which would be extremely difficult for a country dependent on
foreign trade.

In countries unwilling or unable to resort to social surgery,
survival of the population can be achieved only through the
spontaneous adaptation of customs, morals and manners which I
call consuetudinal adaptation. So long as the chances of survival
depend on prudence and self-control, individuals and groups
unendowed with these characteristics will have a much higher
mortality rate which eventually may lead to changes in the
composition of the population. Homosexual inclinations or an
overpowering craving for a variety of sex partners will reduce life
expectancy. The same applies to an inability to form enduring
relationships, the consequence of which is the recurring need to
look for new partners, which entails a higher risk of an unlucky
strike. Promiscuity is perhaps still less common on the middle
rungs of the social ladder than at its extremes: among the
hereditary rich and the subproletariat. The new élite of
entertainers, to repeat, may be wiped out unless it changes its
way of life completely. In contrast, puritanical religious
denominations like the Mormons or the Plymouth Brethren will
thrive. In multi-racial or ethnic societies drastic changes in
numerical proportions may occur in consequence of differences
with respect to promiscuity and prudence. In the USA the
incidence of Aids among the Blacks is four times (and among the
Chicanos two times) higher than among the Whites, while being
substantially lower among people of Asian origin. In Britain
there is censorship of such statistics but the ratios between
corresponding groups are probably very similar.

The Hindu pattern of sexual behaviour is probably best adapted
to survival in the face of Aids. The Hindus marry very early, allow
neither premarital or adulterous affairs and make divorce very
difficult. In contrast to the traditional Catholic pattern, which
prohibits divorce but tolerates adultery (particularly of husbands
with prostitutes), the closed character of a Hindu caste makes
escape from its control almost impossible except in situations where
the entire system is breaking down. The fear of Aids might

revitalise it. I venture a guess that, despite its poverty and insalubrity, India will be less devastated by Aids than most poor non-totalitarian countries.

At the opposite extreme is tropical Africa. Monogamy has no roots there. In the traditional cultures, polygamy was universal, divorce common, premarital copulation and adultery lightly treated, while wives often circulated by being inherited through levirate (the obligation to marry a deceased brother's wife), and similar customs. In the degradation of the cities the few traditional constraints have disappeared and promiscuity is universal. On the top of this, circumcision (especially the atrocious mutilation of girls), rituals of blood brotherhood, decorative scarring and some funeral customs involve the mixing of blood. Hygiene is nonexistent in hospitals (with the exception of the few reserved for the top people) and very rudimentary in doctors' and dentists' surgeries. In any case most extractions of teeth are done by traditional healers, some of whose other treatments also involve contact with blood. There is general trust in the power of injections, which are administered by all kinds of semi-qualified attendants with unsterilised needles. Condoms are unwanted and almost unknown. Information about Aids is either unavailable or disbelieved, while protection against disease is commonly sought in rituals and amulets. It is reported that 20 per cent of the population of Kinshasa and Mombasa is infected. It seems therefore inevitable that the population of Africa will be reduced to a small fraction of its present size.

The prospects are only a little better in other poor countries which are neither Hindu nor Confucian-Communist. Improvidence, promiscuity and prostitution prevail in the slums of Latin America, Indonesia and the Philippines, while compulsive philandering is deeply ingrained in the 'macho' of all classes. Similar attitudes prevail in the Caribbean. The rapid growth of population in these areas will be reversed if Aids continues to spread at the present rate.

A NOTE ON THE ORIGINS

The question of origins remains unsolved. So far, two explanations have been offered. According to some Soviet newspapers, the virus is a product of American preparations for bacteriological warfare. This may be a mere guess or a purely propagandist mendacious assertion. As far as I know, no evidence has been produced. Indeed, it is difficult to see how such a contention could be proved by scientific arguments. The only possible proof would be a secret document obtained by the Soviet espionage from an American research establishment. On the other hand, even if it were true, the relevant authorities would deny it. Moreover, they might know nothing about it because, if the virus escaped by accident, the people responsible for it might have concealed it. Finally, the virus might have escaped accidentally without even the experimenters being aware of it. The main argument against this explanation is that, if a research establishment had had this virus in its laboratory, its scientists would have been the first to unravel its structure once it was in circulation. And they could claim the credit for this discovery without disclosing that they had bred it.

The second explanation is that the Aids virus evolved from the variant which is found in green monkeys. The weakness of this thesis is that it does not explain why this jump across the species barrier took place only recently while the green monkeys have co-existed with mankind for a long time. Many people have eaten green monkeys in the past or (what might be more relevant) have been bitten by them. The same argument applies to the possibility of transmission through sexual abuse: why should this perversion not have been tried before? A possible missing link is supplied by an anthropological report from central Africa written in 1972, but (according to a notice in *The New Scientist*) brought to light in this connection only recently, which mentions the practice of injecting the green monkey's blood into men's veins in the belief that this enhances their sexual prowess. The combination of an ancient superstition with a modern tool for carrying it out constitutes a new situation which might account for a new disease. In contrast, the wide spread of the disease in Africa constitutes no proof that it originated there, because a disease often spreads particularly fast when it is introduced into a new environment, as the examples of syphilis in Europe and smallpox and measles in America show. It is often said that Aids came to America from Africa via Haiti. But why Haiti? There is almost no traffic between Africa and Haiti while there is much between the African capitals and the big American cities – in particular New York. The young members of the Peace Corps and other agencies of US Aid were among the most likely transferrers of Aids in either direction. To the two foregoing hypotheses I would like to add a third. It seems to me that we cannot exclude the possibility that the HIV virus was an accidental (and perhaps unnoticed) by-product of experimentation in genetic engineering, whether for military or pacific purposes. The first ground for my suspicion is that experiments in this field began a little before the putative emergence of Aids. Secondly, when the possibility of genetic engineering was first envisaged, after Crick and Watson discovered the double helix, there appeared in the quality newspapers as well as the science journals letters to the editors from eminent biologists warning against the dangers of unforeseen consequences, in particular of an accidental emergence of a dangerous micro-organism. The third ground for suspicion is that (according to what I read in the *New Scientist* in another context) a virus similar to HIV has been used in experiments aimed at inventing a remedy for some genetic defects. I do not know whether a virus of this type had been used in experiments before the disease struck, but I wonder whether it is altogether impossible in the course of experimentation to cause a mutation (or to help the virus to jump across the species barrier) accidentally or/and indirectly through some kind of chain reactions of micro-organisms on each other. To get the disease going it would have been enough if a single virus entered a single human organism.

If such an origin is not impossible, it may be impossible to ascertain whether an accidential process of this kind has in fact occurred, as it may well have been unobserved. If it had been noticed, it is unlikely that people responsible for it would be eager to come forward to take the blame, particularly if there had been an element of uncertainty in the affair which would have provided a justification for silence. Their fellow specialists would not be particularly eager to pry into this matter because a discrediting revelation might prompt curbs on their own experiments. Moreover, the scientists on the whole (especially the more narrow-minded among them) do not like the idea that research might be directly harmful. And indeed a revelation that a dreadful disease is a direct product of scientific research might provoke a popular reaction against science, leading to revivals of superstition and other flights into irrationality. This would make the survival of mankind even more precarious because a sustainable society – with an economy orientated towards preservation rather than destruction of the environment – will need many inventions and

therefore more rather than less research. We have passed long ago
a point of no return to a pre-scientific way of life.

CONCLUDING REMARKS

On the assumption that the virus becomes neither less nor more
potent, while neither a cure nor a vaccine is invented, we can be
sure that Aids will cause great changes in social life, particularly
in the liberal and open societies not ready to resort to early and
quick medico-social surgery. There can be little doubt that most of
these changes will be very painful – apart from one or two aspects
(like the decline in the illegitimate birth rate) which may be regarded
as improvements on the present way of life. Where neither a
consuetudinal nor socio-surgical adaptation can be carried out, a
massive depopulation will follow.

In the midst of the prospect there is only one possible consolation:
that this dreadful calamity may forestall something even worse.
Though bringing upon mankind terrible sufferings, the Aids virus
in its present form does not threaten the survival of our species.
We can be certain that, no matter how many may die, many others
will take sufficient precautions to escape infection and perpetuate
the species. In contrast, no one – no matter how prudent and
ingenious – can escape the ecological calamities looming on the
not-so-distant horizon. If we assume that present trends will
continue, and extrapolate the rates of accumulation of radioactive
materials, the depletion of the ozone layer, the decrease in production of oxygen in consequence of the destruction of plant life, the
greenhouse effect, and other kinds of lethal pollution, then the
inference follows that mankind does not have a long future before
it.

These calamitous trends result mainly from two sets of circumstances: overpopulation, and the antisocial wastrel's attitude to the
resources of our planet, which implies a total lack of concern
for future generations and rests upon a crazy disregard of the
indubitable fact that the earth is round and therefore incapable of
accommodating an indefinite compound growth of anything. It is
perhaps too much to hope that the shock of Aids may shake
mankind out of the drunken vandal's attitude to the environment,
although it is not altogether impossible that the enforced individual
prudence might attenuate the collective improvidence. It is very

likely, however, that Aids will put an end to the population explosion. If mankind does not have enough wisdom to avert the ecological catastrophe in a less painful way, depopulation caused by Aids might be the lesser evil.

Notes

1. The weakness of this assumption is that it is unproven. Given that there are racial differences in vulnerability to some diseases, it is not impossible that this might also be the case with Aids. However, it is difficult to ascertain this, since the present spread of the infection appears to be explicable by environmental factors.
2. I prefer 'immunity system' to the usual term 'immune system' which is illogical because it is not really immune itself. If it were, Aids could not exist. The best term is 'the defence system' because it does defend the organism, though the immunity to infections which it provides is strictly limited and often insufficient.
3. Since this was written the government has introduced a price differential to encourage the use of lead-free petrol.

Appendix Two

Wickedness, Madness and Error: on the Limits of the Usefulness of Psychoanalysis in Historical Explanation

The works of Sigmund Freud constitute one of the greatest feats of inquiring imagination ever accomplished: they enlarged our intellectual horizon by an entire battery of new concepts which have changed fundamentally our way of thinking about human nature and conduct. This, however, does not mean that they are free from very serious errors which sometimes go to the point of absurdity. Furthermore, although he must be admired for the extraordinary fertility of his intellect, we must bear in mind that, like every other genius, he built upon the work of his predecessors and contemporaries. The dogmatism of 'the Freudians' (only a little less silly than that of the Marxists) ought not to deter us from trying to make the best use of Freud's bequest by discarding the errors and exaggerations, and following the valid insights which enable us to explain a number of aspects of human behaviour which otherwise remain completely inexplicable. Since he was the first to offer any kind of explanation for a number of neuroses and since his explanations were in terms of the workings of the sexual instinct, it is understandable that in the flush of excitement he was inclined to push his theories beyond reasonable bounds and tried to explain everything along these lines. However, Freud's ideas about unconscious motivation, the mechanisms of symptom formation, and treatment do not depend on pansexualism, that is the paradigm of tracing everything to sexual desire. Already at the beginnings of psychoanalysis, one of Freud's disciples, Alfred Adler, developed a theory which incorporated Freud's concepts of unconscious goal-seeking, repression of thoughts from the field of consciousness, projection, ambivalence and so on, but which made the quest for power and admiration into the dominant motive of human behaviour. Slightly later, William MacDougall interpreted the workings of the instinct of self-preservation in the light of Freud's concepts of mental mechanisms, and he even applied the latter's methods of therapy (analysis and abreaction) in the treatment of 'war neuroses'. Working as a psychiatrist in the British Army hospitals during the First World War, MacDougall had to deal with patients who experienced extreme and well-justified fear, unlike Freud's patients who were safe physically and financially, and had plenty of time to think mainly about sex. MacDougall made an interesting discovery: that many cases of disability labelled as shell shock were due not so much to fear itself as to the repression thereof from the consciousness. He found that shell shock was less common among the French soldiers, and explains this difference in his *Outline of Abnormal Psychology* (1926) by saying that they were less inclined to repress fear from the field of consciousness because they were more open about admitting that they had been scared, whereas the British soldiers, indoctrinated with the cult of 'the stiff upper lip', more often denied it. By applying the Freudian method of abreaction – that is, leading his patients to recall and re-live their frightening experiences – MacDougall was able in many cases (he does not say how many) to cure such symptoms of shell shock as paralysis of the limbs, inability to speak, or dizziness.

We can see thus that already at the beginning of psychoanalysis Freud's theories have been modified by limitation as well as extension: his pansexualism was rejected but his ideas of mental mechanisms of censorship, repression, complex and symptom formation, projection, ambivalence and unconscious goal-seeking or strategy, have been applied to instincts other than the sexual. By instinct I mean a genetically determined propensity, universal in the species and necessary to its survival.) Adler has certainly exaggerated the importance of the desire for power by mixing it up with the desire for social acceptance and approval. The latter can be called an instinct, as defined above: we are a social species and not even our simian ancestors could have survived as solitary animals. In contrast the desire for power is a common but not a universal propensity. Although Freud talks about libido (the all-pervasive sexual instinct) as the only universal driving force, his concepts of the censor and the superego presuppose the existence of another motive of equal universality: for whence would the censor and the superego draw the force needed to constrain the libido and to drive libidinous thoughts out of the field of consciousness (to repress them, in his terminology) if not from the need for social acceptance and approval? There is plenty of evidence to show that the lack of (or insecurity about) the satisfaction of this need can produce neuroses just as severe as various sexual hangups. Anyway, the workings of these two propensities are often inextricably mixed.

There has been much discussion about the uses of psychoanalysis in interpreting historical events and personalities, but the attempts to do so in concrete cases have brought little that can be regarded as acceptably solid knowledge. One reason for this is the weakness which the authors of such interpretations share with most historians, who are very careful about ascertaining what happened but cavalier – indeed often downright slapdash – in their assertions about why it happened. Within the traditional limits of their craft the historians can hardly remedy this fault except by avoiding explanations, and sticking to a straightforward account of the facts, because an explanatory thesis cannot emerge from a narrative no matter how detailed, except through unwarranted jumping from 'after' to 'because' (*post hoc ergo propter hoc*). Support for a surmisal of a causal connection between historical processes can only be obtained through comparative analysis which might show co-variation or some approximation to Mill's inductive canons of agreement or difference.

Given the complexity of the phenomena and the impossibility of experimentation, no historical explanation can attain the standards of confirmation expected in the exact sciences. We must bear in mind the canons of methodological perfection but insistence on unattainable standards must lead to sterility. Historical and sociological explanations and theories must move on the intermediate level between bare assertion and conclusive proof. Seeking an explanation, we have to search for pointers, each of which is inconclusive alone but adds a little to the credibility of the others until we can accumulate a logically consistent set which makes the thesis highly likely to be true. Fitting the pointers together, we can make use of indirect arguments, such as the absence of evidence supporting the negation of the thesis. For instance, in addition to the evidence of positive co-variation we can ask whether there are any reasons for believing that the epidemic of syphilis could not have caused the fear of witches. We can also start at the other end and ask whether an epidemic which is known to have wrought great havoc and panic was likely to pass without causing important changes in the social life. And if we judge that this was very unlikely, we can take the next step and ask which aspects of life might have been affected. Given the nature of the disease, it seems prima facie likely that it would have had a great impact on the attitudes to sexual pleasures and of the sexes to one another.

Except when we are asking a very commonplace question like 'why are they hungry?' there is little room in the study of human societies for the classic 'covering law' model of explanation, where a phenomenon P is said to be explained by a statement of the initial condition C and of a covering law L (that is, a well-established generalisation) according to which C is always followed by P. There are very few general propositions in the social sciences whose truth can be taken for granted; but if we find that the data fit a given proposition, we can draw the conclusion that the likelihood of it being true is thereby enhanced. Very seldom can we take any generalisation as proven beyond doubt. Even those ideas of psychoanalysis which appear to be best confirmed by observation do not belong among the most securely established propositions of the social sciences. Consequently, there ought to be no question of accepting an explanation which merely cites one of them as a covering law. In view of their tenuousness, we must have other evidence of the existence of the causal link which psychoanalysis makes understandable or enables us to surmise. As far as historical explanation is concerned, such evidence can only be supplied by comparative analysis, which is absent from the efforts hitherto made to explain history or contemporary political situations by psychoanalysis. Let us look at an example which shows how an explanatory thesis backed by massive though rather ethnocentric erudition can be refuted as soon as we look at it from a comparative viewpoint.

In an interesting collection of essays published in Paris in 1937 under the title *Autorität und Familie*, written by German Jewish refugee scholars who were acquainted with history as well as psychoanalysis, the recurrent theme is that the authoritarian (to be precise, patriarchal) structure of the German family explains Nazism. However, the argument rests either on deduction from psychoanalytic theory or on an inference from co-existence to causation. No question is raised whether the rise of the Nazi movement was preceded or accompanied by an intensification of the patriarchy in Germany. Unfortunately for the thesis, the facts point to an opposite conclusion: patriarchy was much weaker in 1933 than in 1833 when German nationalists strove for liberalism and parliamentarianism. Although the German family in the nineteen-thirties may have been a little more authoritarian than the English family at that time, it was much less so than the Victorian family. Actually, a more plausible case could be made for the view that a decline of patriarchy constituted a precondition of the rise of mass movements, recruiting and moulding young men and women often against the wishes of their parents. Although the Italian family was fairly patriarchal at the time of Mussolini's triumph, it was considerably less so than in the days of Garibaldi. Between the wars, patriarchy seems to have been stronger in Italy than in Germany, and may have played a role in preventing the Fascists from being as successful as the Nazis in moulding the youth. The first error of the thesis in question consists of attempting to explain something recent and local (Fascism and Nazism) by a factor (authoritarian patriarchy) which is much older and more widespread – indeed prevalent throughout the world.

It is a common error to push a useful explanatory scheme beyond the limits of its validity. Psychoanalysis offers a key to certain doors for which no other key is at present available. We should not be put off from using it by the antics of doctrinaires who regard it as a magic key to all the mysteries and make it into a religion. Social changes can occur without a prior or accompanying change in the motivation. Prices, for instance, can move up or down without any change in the dealers' desire to buy cheap and sell dear. A conquest may take place because an invention gives one side a relative superiority and victory without any change in the martial propensities or virtues.

Since only among German Jews were to be found people who knew about psychoanalysis as well as history – and since they were naturally deeply upset and perplexed by the disaster – a preoccupation with the phenomenon of Nazism pervaded the attempts to make use of psychoanalysis in historical explanation. This was unfortunate from a scientific viewpoint because of the importance in this case of factors which do not come within the horizon of psychoanalysis. A search for causes connected with patterns of sex life brought to light nothing convincing.

In their sexual habits, the pattern of relationships between the sexes or the treatment of children, the Germans did not differ radically from other European nations, and so it is very farfetched to argue, as the psychoanalysts Reich and Reik do, that the rise of the Nazi movement can be linked to sexual frustration, particularly since the Nazis fostered a relaxation of sexual morals and a disregard for the Christian ideal of premarital chastity. Nor shall we get very far towards an explanation of the mass movement by searching for sexual kinks among the Nazi leaders. Firstly because there are kinky men in all countries, and there is no evidence that they were more abundant in Germany than anywhere else. So, even if we could prove that all the Nazi leaders had sexual kinks, the question would still remain why people of this type won power in Germany and not in other countries. This question, however, hardly arises, because there is no evidence that Hitler and his cronies engaged in any extraordinary sexual practices. Roehm, Heydrich and a few others were homosexuals, but the percentage of the latter seems to have been lower among the Nazis than among the British politicians. It may be distressing but it is a fact that in their private lives the Nazi leaders were very ordinary men, with tastes typical of the lower middle class. The only truly extraordinary characteristic of Hitler was his genius for demagoguery – as a rabble-rouser he had no rival in recent European history. It is a common inclination to revile enemies by attributing to them sexual abnormalities regardless of the truth.

Although people who volunteered for manning the concentration camps were self-selected for sadism or at least extreme callousness, none of the top Nazi chiefs carried out acts of killing or torturing personally. Unlike the founder of the Soviet police – the syphilitic Polish squire Felix Dzierzynski – who personally shot hundreds, if not thousands, Himmler is known to have hit someone only once, while nothing of this kind is recorded of Hitler or Goebbels. Eichmann seems to have been a mere soulless bureaucrat who did what he was told: he obviously had no great moral objections to organising a mass slaughter but there is no evidence that he particularly relished it. We may well suspect that Hitler and Himmler did enjoy issuing orders condemning millions to death but their sadism was not so direct as that of many Roman emperors. In the Roman circuses, when a gladiator was about to cut the throat of his defeated opponent, he had to turn the latter's face towards the imperial stand so that the Emperor and his guests could see the expression on the victim's face. The annals of history are full of records of bloody deeds, and if we insisted that they all must have stemmed from madness, then we would have to classify most of the rulers of the past as lunatics.

Although sexual frustration and repression may prompt certain kinds of cruelty, there are ample proofs that total disregard of human life, cruelty and even obvious sadism need not stem from this source, as the aforementioned examples of the Roman emperors suffice to show. Nor did the sultans suffer from the lack of carnal pleasures . . . which did not prevent them chopping off heads with great alacrity. To relieve overcrowding of their harems, some of them used to order the slaughter of a part of their inmates. In his courageous book *Purdah and Polygamy* (Karachi: Readers Associates, 1972, p. 49), the Pakistani author Mazhar Ul Haq Khan writes:

Countless women were killed by irate husbands and irascible masters all over the Muslim world in the Middle Ages, but the Ottoman Turks proved to be the cruellest in this respect. Their usual technique of disposing of an unfaithful or unwanted wife or woman was to sew her up in a sack and throw her into a well, stream, river or sea nearby, to be drowned to death. Writing of the Imperial harems of the Ottoman Sultans, N. M. Penzer says, 'The drowning of one or two women would attract no notice at all, and everything would be carried out with silence and dispatch. The Kislar Agha takes them to the Bostanji-bashi, under whose direction the hapless females are placed in sacks weighted with stones. The bostanji, to whom the duty of drowning them is committed, board a small rowing-boat to which is attached by a rope a smaller one in which the women are placed. They then row towards the open water opposite Seraglio point, and by several dexterous jerks of the rope cause the boat to capsize. A eunuch accompanies the bostanji and reports to the Kislar Agha the fulfilment of his orders.

At times, however, a mass drowning would take place on the discovery of some plot to depose the Sultan or similar grave offence. As many as 300 women have been drowned on such an occasion. The most terrible case was during the reign of Ibrahim (1640–48), who after one of his debauches suddenly decided to drown his complete harem just for the fun of getting a new one later on. Accordingly several hundred women were seized, and thrown into the Bosphorus. Only one escaped. She was picked up by a passing vessel and ultimately reached Paris.

A psychoanalytic explanation of such cruelty must follow the lines foreshadowed by MacDougall rather than Freud; seeing it as a reaction to having grown up under the menace of violent death. The young princes had unlimited opportunities for sexual indulgence but they lived in a world of murderous intrigues and fear, and they had to inhibit every impulse to love and trust. They could not even trust their own mother if she had more than one son because the rule was that upon ascending the throne the new sultan would kill not only all his half-brothers but full brothers as well. There was a special platoon of deaf-mutes always ready for the task of strangling the princes with bowstrings. It is difficult to understand how a man could have issued a decree which condemned all his sons but one to death, and how his successors could bear maintaining it for many generations, but we certainly cannot explain it by postulating a repression of sexual desires on their part.

With their concept of sadism, psychoanalysts have overgeneralised: from the undoubted fact that in some individuals sexual pleasure gets mixed up with the enjoyment derived from inflicting pain or death, they inferred that it must always be so. However, there are innumerable examples of killing and cruelty where there are no traces of sexual excitement: the pleasure which the perpetrators derive seems to be linked with the enjoyment of power. The clearest demonstration of power is to be able to do to someone something which they most dislike. If we are to retain the term 'sadism' for any kind of enjoyment of cruelty, we ought to distinguish sexual sadism from non-sexual, connected with the lust for power. We must also bear in mind that not always is pain inflicted for the sake of the pleasure derived from doing so. Much cruelty is instrumental – that is, used as a means to an end. The attitude accompanying its perpetration is often sheer indifference or callousness rather than delight. There is no evidence that Napoleon, for example, positively enjoyed other people's sufferings: he seems to have been merely indifferent to them and was always ready to sacrifice other men's lives in pursuit of his ambitions. The dreadful deeds of Stalin also appear as the means to his ends. Like Hitler, Stalin never personally witnessed the grisly proceedings which he set in motion. There is no record of him exulting about the atrocities perpetrated on his orders. Joyless callousness seems to have been his characteristic: it is evident that he was totally indifferent to the sufferings of others and felt no greater compunction about sending people to death than most of us feel about killing a mosquito. Nor are there grounds for attributing to him paranoia. True, he was extremely suspicious, always on the lookout for plots, and he took great precautions against being assassinated or poisoned; but he had very good reasons for his fear, having murdered so many people during his climb to the top. But why did he resort to murder in the first place? The answer is that he could not become the absolute master of the Kremlin except by intrigue, intimidation and murder, because he was not highly regarded by other prominent leaders of the Revolution. Furthermore, since his rule was contrary to the ideals of the Revolution, he had to eliminate all those who took them seriously. Even the mass purges, in which many of his obedient servants perished, were not crazy witch hunts but a rational (though terribly wicked) method of establishing total power. This method was based on two assumptions:

(1) That it is safer to kill many innocent people than to let one enemy escape.
(2) That resistance is most effectively paralysed, and unquestioning obedience induced, by all-pervading fear.

Collectivisation of the agriculture (which caused the death of several million peasants) may have been a mistake but this is not certain, as there may have been no faster method of building up the heavy armaments industries. To concentrate resources in those fields it was necessary to neglect the production of consumption goods, so that there was nothing to offer to the peasants to induce them to produce and sell the food needed to feed the rapidly growing mass of industrial workers and bureaucrats, not to speak of the army and the police. So an extension of state slavery to agriculture was a logical step.

All Stalin's actions can be seen as rational steps towards his goals, pursued with a total disregard of ethical considerations. Of all the leaders in the Second World War, Stalin was the only true winner. Roosevelt and Truman failed to achieve their goal of making the world safe for ever for the Americans, while Churchill was a complete failure (in relation to the values which he professed), who led his country to a defeat disguised as a victory. Britain went to war not for the love of Poland but to prevent the formation in central Europe of a dangerous military empire. Britain's 'victory', however, helped to establish in that area an even more dangerous empire. Churchill declared many times that his aim was to preserve the British Empire but he helped to produce a situation in which it had to be dismantled, as Britain became unable to defend even its own independence (not to speak of the Empire) without American protection. In his enthusiasm for knocking down the foe, intoxicated by his own oratory and perhaps with his mind weakened by dependence on alcohol, Churchill handed over to Stalin more than what was denied to Hitler at the price of six years of devastation and carnage. In contrast, Stalin was a moral monster but, as a political strategist and tactician, a genius of the first order. To see him as mad amounts to mere wishful thinking.

The habit of dubbing as mad everybody who (or every action which) is bad constitutes a part of the general climate of euphemism and avoidance of unpleasant truths which pervades our culture, and which has prompted the renaming of countless conditions and institutions: the old have become 'middle-aged'; mental defectives have become 'retarded' although they will never catch up; Sick Rooms have become Health Centres although no healthy people go there; countries which are sinking into every greater misery are called 'developing'; being interrogated in prison is referred to on the radio and in the newspapers as 'helping the police with their enquiries', while (to end with the silliest example) the poor have been renamed 'underprivileged' – which term carries the nonsensical implication that everybody could be privileged. Denying that normal people can be wicked may be a comforting belief, but it is contrary to the facts unless we make it true by definition and take the commission of a cruel deed as evidence of insanity. This is often done: many people say that the Yorkshire Ripper must be mad because otherwise he would have not done what he has. However, he has shown no other signs of madness apart from his taste for mutilating and killing women, and while pursuing this hobby he took perfectly rational steps to cover up his tracks. True, he took a risk but no greater than what many sportsmen are prepared to face. His predecessor was never caught. Many of the Nazi butchers and torturers who managed to hide themselves lived for many years as ordinary people, unsuspected by their neighbours, until chance brought them face to face with one of their victims. They gave an impression of being ordinary, perfectly decent (in some cases even nice) individuals. Since people like the Yorkshire Ripper take considerable risks, we can presume that they derive great pleasure from their deeds. The Nazi prison guards did not think there was any danger in it, so we do not know how many of them took delight in tormenting and killing people, and how many were merely callous and saw it as an easy way of making a living, or of avoiding the more dangerous service at the front.

In their book *Power and Morality* (Boston: Porter Sargent, 1959), Pitirim Sorokin and Walter Lunde present the results of their enquiry into the crimes committed by absolute rulers in the past. They exclude political crimes which could not be committed by ordinary people and count only such acts as the murder of a relative or friend, incest, rape or the unlawful seizure of property for one's personal use. On their estimate, the royal dynasties constitute the true criminal class, with crime rates many times higher than among ordinary people. This does not prove that their inclinations were much worse than those of ordinary folk, albeit this might have been so, because the difference may be explained by the fact that they had much ampler opportunities for giving vent to their proclivities with impunity.

There are innumerable examples of cruel practices carried out as a means to an end: usually an appropriation of other people's work or possessions. Slavery and serfdom offered wide opportunities to sadists to indulge their proclivities but the common aim of all the masters was exploitation. Many of them resorted to chaining, whipping, branding and crucifying, not for the pleasure of it, but to enforce obedience and make the slaves work for them, so that they would not have to work themselves. At the level of productivity which prevailed before machines were invented it was impossible to acquire wealth through one's own productive work, and so nobody could live in affluence without being a party to exploitation backed by cruel coercion. As the desire for living in comfort is universal (apart from a few ascetics), there is no need to search for hidden motives with the aid of psychoanalysis to explain the cruel treatment of the poor. In a Roman textbook of estate management the author discusses the question of the age at which a slave's output falls below the cost of upkeep so that it becomes advisable to kill him or her. There is no trace of sadism in what he says: the tone is perfectly matter-of-fact and businesslike, similar to what you find in present day publications for farmers when they talk about the cattle.

Hitler was less clever than Stalin and made more serious errors. He also seems to have believed more genuinely in his doctrine and was less ready to bend it for the sake of a tactical advantage. He was a liar in day-to-day tactics, but as far as the doctrine was concerned, his level of sincerity seems to have been nearer to that of Lenin and Trotsky rather than Stalin. It was his and his cronies' devotion to the doctrine of the racial inferiority of the Slavs that led them to throw away the opportunity of a victory over the USSR by obtaining the support of the Russian and Ukrainian people against their rulers. He made a number of other mistakes in his campaign but they were no worse than Napoleon's decision to march on Moscow. Had he been cleverer, he might have used anti-Semitism to hoist himself to power, but afterwards he would have used the enormous brainpower and patriotism of the German Jews instead of driving them out or killing them. Even without the Jewish scientists, he might have had an atomic bomb in 1944 had he organised a proper effort. He could have easily forced Franco to join him, could have seized Gibraltar and sealed off the access to the Mediterranean. All these mistakes, however, do not add up to madness: they were not more absurd than thousands of decisions of other rulers which by hindsight we can see as mistaken.

Indeed, no mistake of Hitler was as silly as what Roosevelt did at the end of the Second World War when, despite being in a much stronger position, he gave Stalin (of whose enmity and ferocity there was plenty of evidence) half of Europe, Manchuria, half of Korea and a bit of Japan. Even Hitler's most irrational act – the declaration of war against the United States – was not quite so silly, as he was gambling on inducing thereby Japan to attack the USSR, which might have prevented his defeat at Stalingrad. The diversion of resources to the extermination of the Jews, or the razing of Warsaw to the ground, were of course acts of great wickedness but not particularly irrational, because by then Hitler knew that he had lost the war and that the diversion of resources for the purpose of giving vent to his venom would make no difference to the outcome. We must also bear in mind that the deeds of the Nazis were a shocking relapse into barbarity only in relation to the standards of civilised behaviour which developed in Europe during the eighteenth and nineteenth centuries. In comparison with the wars and conquests of earlier times (or with some events which occurred more recently outside Europe, like the extermination of most of the Armenians in the Ottoman empire during the First World War), there was nothing extraordinary about the Nazi atrocities except their mechanisation. Their dreadful treatment of the Poles and the Russians, or even the Jews, was no worse than that of the Albigensians by Simon de Montfort, of the Carthaginians by Scipio Africanus, or of the Persians by Hulagu, the Mongol conqueror. More often than not the defeated had only the choice between death (often very cruel) or the chains of slavery in the literal sense of the word. So, if we take perpetration of atrocity as a proof of insanity, we have to conclude that sanity is abnormal in the sense of being historically rare.

Calling 'mad' everybody who is bad may satisfy the bent for wishful thinking but it does not lead to improved understanding and, therefore, cannot help to prevent suffering, because no prophylactic can succeed (except by sheer chance) if it is based on a false diagnosis of causes. Likewise, employing psychiatry wantonly to vilify the enemy (or to make him appear less formidable) is likely to prompt unwise strategy. Irrational actions, that is, actions which are absurdly futile, self-defeating or counter-productive in relation to the doer's goals, characterise (nay, define) neurotic behaviour; but it is seldom easy to distinguish between irrationality and error due to inadequate knowledge. Consequently if we want to use psychoanalysis in historical and sociological explanation, we must look for patterns of behaviour which can be regarded neither as the means to a given end (that is, as rationally instrumental actions) nor as unintended consequences of such rationally instrumental actions, nor as being prompted by a simple habit persisting through the force of sheer mental inertia. Furthermore, if we wish to rely on Freud's own ideas, we must look for patterns of behaviour which might have something to do with the workings of the sexual instinct. It is no use expecting psychoanalysis to help us to explain the Great Crash on the Stock Exchange, whereas the all-pervading fear of witches and the puritanical shunning of all pleasures call for an explanation which makes use of Freud's ideas.

Even a genius can be very wrong, and such an approach in no way entails an acceptance of all Freud's theories, not to speak of his misfired historical explanations which represent the very nadir of his work. Though not quite so daft as the notions of some of his crazy disciples – one of which attributes capitalism to anal eroticism while another explains religion by onanism – Freud's explanation of totemism and taboo is on the same intellectual level as explaining human aggressiveness and war by the deed of Cain. Disregarding the ethnographic evidence, Freud assumes the universality of totemism in primitive societies, and then proceeds to explain it by a single event of which there can be no evidence: namely, a fictitious case of a rebellion in a prehistoric horde where the sons killed the patriarch, ate him, and then repressed their feelings of guilt which compelled them to go on propitiating his ghost.

Although he never descends to this level of crudity in his proper field, many of his psychological views were also wrong. As many anthropologists (beginning with Malinowski in the nineteen-twenties) have shown, one of the most important sources of errors was the taking for granted that the small sector of the Viennese society whence his patients came represented a universal pattern of interpersonal relations. Some of his open-minded followers – most notably Erich Fromm and Karen Horney – corrected this shortcoming by taking into account cultural variations. Further-more, although it was a brilliantly fruitful idea to play down the frontier between the sane and the insane, and to look at human nature in the light of psychopathology, Freud overshoots the mark and more or less disregards the difference. Despite his marvellously original insights into the etiology and symptoms of neuroses, as well as into mental processes in general, he provides no answer to the question of why some people go mad or neurotic while others don't. This is not surprising, because (except when he deals with jokes and mistakes) all his data come from observing his or his colleagues' patients. He does not consider the possibility that because of a more balanced mental constitution, the people who never needed a psychiatrist may not have suffered from an Oedipus complex, penis envy, fear of castration, a predilection for faeces or any of the other tendencies which he found at the root of his patients' illnesses.

Fortunately Freud's ideas about mental mechanisms – such as repression, projection and so on – depend neither on the aforementioned shortcomings nor on his unwarranted unilinear theory of stages of mental development or the pansexualism. The first can be very useful for explaining history but we must avoid unsupported assertion which marred most (if not all) attempts in this direction. The methodological rule which I have tried to follow here can be likened to a two-pronged attack: a co-variation between mass phenomena must be established (or at least supported) by a comparative analysis of historical ethnographic or sociographic data, while the nature of the link between them is illuminated by psycho-analytic (or other psychological) theory derived from observations of individual behaviour in other (but somewhat parallel) situations. Since it is unlikely that the results of the two approaches might mesh in by sheer chance, the fact of them fitting together enhances the likelihood of each of them being valid.

Postscript February 1989

Since the foregoing forecast was written more than a year ago, a few supplementary points have occurred to me and some new information and arguments have reached me which call for comments. This applies in the first place to the interesting book by Gene Antonio, *The Aids Cover Up?*[1].

Despite the question mark in the title, Antonio has no doubt that the politicians and medical authorities are concealing the magnitude of the danger because they do not want to do anything about it. He makes a convincing case. As I have not observed the American scene with equal thoroughness, I cannot judge whether all his accusations are justified, but I think he is right on the whole. One of my reasons for thinking so is that we can observe an analogous phenomenon in Britain.

The desire not to know is not merely accompanied by the reluctance to act, but largely stems from it. The reason for this reluctance is that any kind of action will offend one or another influential circle. Broadly speaking these circles fall into two camps. On one side are various religious congregations (as well as the less religious upholders of the traditional values) who are deeply offended by the propaganda in favour of 'safe sex', which publicly advocates condoms and openly discusses the sexual practices which until recently were treated as abhorrent and unmentionable in decent company. On the other side are the ultra-permissive liberals, ready to defend anyone's right to 'do his own thing' regardless of the consequences for others. They are vaguely allied with the homosexual circles.

This camp is in favour of the propaganda (or education, if you prefer) for 'safe sex' – in fact they complain that there is not enough of it – but they vehemently oppose any proposals to protect the uninfected at the price of making the life of the infected unpleasant. The more devoutly religious pressure groups are less concerned about the welfare of the infected, whose condition they view as 'the wages of sin'; apart from the interment of the carriers, the only remedial action of which they approve is the stepping up of preaching against sin. The obvious impossibility of satisfying both camps largely accounts for the vacillation of the politicians, the medical authorities and the controllers of the media.

In the USA the permissivist camp is strong, while the homosexual lobby is well-organised and active. But the militant religious congregations are even stronger. The resulting stalemate makes inaction almost inevitable.

In Britain the strength of the permissivist camp (including its homosexual wing) is greater than that of militant religious bodies, mainly because the Church of England has become very liberal and tepid in matters of faith. Consequently, the government and the medical authorities have been ready to offend the traditional sense of morality and propriety by launching a campaign for 'safe sex', but have studiously avoided any steps which might cause suffering or even merely an inconvenience to the infected. The best example is the question of anonymous testing. The doctors, who might test their patients without consent, have been threatened with prosecution for assault. This attitude is inexplicable except by a positive desire for ignorance. For what kind of 'assault' is it to have a few drops of blood taken painlessly? It is said that being tested without consent constitutes an infringement of freedom. But how can an operation which takes a few seconds, is painless and leaves no traces diminish your freedom? Certainly much less than being obliged to put on a seat-belt. The absurdity of this notion is even more evident when we bear in mind that in most cases it would not be necessary to take blood especially for this purpose, as most patients in hospitals have blood tests anyway.

Even compulsory and communicated testing would be at least as justifiable as breathalysing. After all, there can be no more basic right than to put into one's mouth whatever one likes. Yet this right is restricted when its exercise affects adversely the safety of others. As a general principle, I have the right to avoid unpleasant truth so long as my ignorance does not endanger others. It is very distressing to hear that one, fairly mild, complaint is the first sign of, say, Parkinson's or Alzheimer's disease. Ignorance is by far a happier condition. But no one argues that a pilot or even a mere ordinary driver has the right to happiness on such a basis. Why should such a right be vouchsafed to a carrier of Aids? Why should his or her right to peace of mind through ignorance be rated as more important than the right of others not to be exposed to a deadly infection?

Nobody (as far as I know) has explicitly asserted that the right of a carrier to enjoyment through ignorance is more important than the safety of others. The usual stance of the advocates of inaction is never to acknowledge that the two rights are incompatible. According to a report in the *Independent*:

Doctors who test patients for Aids without their knowledge or consent must be prepared to defend their decision in court or before their disciplinary body, the British Medical Association decided yesterday.

Tests should only take place on clinical grounds, and with the consent of the patient, the association's annual meeting in Norwich decided.

The decision largely reverses the call by last year's annual meeting for doctors to be allowed to test patients without necessarily seeking their consent. Hospital doctors at last year's meeting argued that it was necessary to protect themselves, their staff and their families.

That decision, however, was criticised by Aids specialists who warned that secret testing would drive the disease underground.

So it seems that the British Medical Association disregards the right of the healthy not to be exposed to avoidable risks. This is rather surprising, particularly as the argument about 'the underground' is nonsensical if not disingenuous. What is this 'underground'? Where is it? The only possible meaning that we can attach to 'going underground' is 'keeping away from doctors', which would be difficult for people who need medical help. In any case, even if they did, what difference would it make, given that the doctors can neither cure them nor reduce their infectiousness? Anyway what can the carriers do 'underground' which they would not be doing 'overground' when, infected but untested, they copulate happily with uninfected partners?

A member of the association's council (according to the same report) said that

'if a patient who had had a fling abroad came to the doctor with vague symptoms and the doctor told him that he was to be tested for Aids the man might be devastated,' he said. 'He goes home and his wife takes one look at his face and asks him what is wrong. He says he might have Aids and his wife says: "But that's impossible . . . isn't it?" He tells all.

'He comes back to you five days later and is told: "Great news. The test is negative." It might be great news for you, he says, but his marriage is over. It is bad medicine to alarm the patient unnecessarily.'

So, according to this version of medical ethics, the most important consideration in such a situation is not to cause a liar to be found out . . . it is much better to risk the health and life of an innocent woman.

The report ends by saying: 'If doctors undertook tests to try to protect themselves or their staff they would, on the BMA's legal advice, be outside the law.'

There is no mention of any justification for denying to people the right not to be exposed to avoidable risks of infection. A necessary corollary of this right is that no one has the right to impose such risks on others because of his or her desire not to face a painful truth about his or her condition. If follows that it would be fair to make willingness to be tested a condition of receiving medical care or being allowed to work in it.

It is impossible to think of a convincing justification for the reluctance to declare Aids to be a notifiable disease like some which are less dangerous. In Britain the general practitioners have been instructed that if they find out that a patient has Aids but refuses to tell his wife, they must keep the secret. It is true that confidentiality in a doctor-patient relationship is a very valuable custom. But every worthy principle can be pushed to absurd lengths, as here to the point of requiring the doctor to be an accomplice in a crime. For it is surely better to murder somebody quickly than to infect them with an illness which first causes a long period of mental torment, then a shorter but still quite long period of suffering and finally a slow and painful death. If a madman tells his doctor that he hears voices which tell him to strangle his wife, he will be locked up in an asylum. So, why should carriers of Aids have a licence to kill? And why should their doctors be expected to connive? It is true that the partner may escape infection, and that the carrier may not copulate for the purpose of infecting him or her. In such a case a more exact analogy would be a motor mechanic who for the sake of his convenience or profit (or merely to cover up his shortcomings) conceals from the customer that the steering is faulty and may jam any moment. The law treats such a concealment as a crime (provided, of course that it can be proved) even if the customer discovers it before an accident occurs. Anybody who connived with such a concealment would also be liable to prosecution. In Germany people have been sent to prison for knowingly infecting another person with Aids. Nobody has been prosecuted for such an offence in Britain, but it would be an interesting case if someone started a private prosecution either against the infector who concealed his or her condition or the doctor who connived with this concealment. The doctor could also be sued under the civil law for damages. If no rational clarification of the law is undertaken in this matter, the doctors may find themselves under fire from both ends.

It is very likely that the hospitals will be forced by lawsuits to test their personnel because, if a patient catches Aids from another member of the staff through some kind of contact with body fluids – which is more likely in such a situation than in an office, shop or even restaurant – the plaintiff could argue that exposing him or her to such a risk amounted to culpable negligence, because the hospital possessed the means to prevent it. Such suits would be complicated and costly because of the difficulty of proving or refuting the claims. The hospitals might find it prudent to test everyone on admission as well as their personnel.

If it is true, as Gene Antonio argues, that the homosexual lobby is responsible for the resistance against testing, then they are unwise and short-sighted. One can sympathise with their fear of persecution, but this is particularly likely to occur if a prolonged ostrich-like attitude suddenly gives way to a panic. A gradual and rational adaptation is much less likely to lead to wild outbursts of scapegoating. However, although there is no doubt a good deal of truth in what he says, I think Antonio goes too far in attributing the predilection for inaction entirely to the influence of the homosexual lobby. One reason why this explanation appears to be only partial is that the tendency to avoid unpleasant truths and postpone costly remedies can be seen in connection with other dangers (especially the ecological) which are even graver than Aids. The ostrich-like attitude (to use the expression unfair to ostriches who bury their heads in the sand merely to avoid heat), is especially striking on the question of overpopulation, which can be understood with no knowledge of science or the need to rely on the opinions of experts, as anyone who can calculate compound growth can verify that the present rate of growth is not sustainable: within a few centuries there would be no room for everyone to stand, even if the oceans were covered with platforms. High fertility can co-exist with low mortality only during short periods in exceptionally favourable circumstances. Otherwise birth and death rates must oscillate around equality. For example, if the death rate in Ethiopia were brought down to West-European level while the birth rate remained what it is now, then within 98 years there would be more Ethiopians than there are people in the world today. It follows that no attempt to improve the living conditions in a poor country with a high birth rate can succeed without birth control. Yet this obvious fact is assiduously concealed. There is in fact an informal censorship in this matter, exercised by the editors of newspapers and broadcasts, with the result that this fundamental problem is very seldom mentioned and never properly discussed.

The inclination to disregard dangers which cannot be seen but only inferred through abstract reasoning, is a common human characteristic. But it is aggravated by some features of the political game. To succeed in it is such hard work that sufficient persistence is most often prompted by a craving for power. In an ideal society, such motivation would disqualify a candidate. Moreover, the struggle for power (whether to get it or to hold it) is so absorbing that many (perhaps most) politicians can hardly think of anything else. Furthermore, the skill of getting or retaining power does not entail the knowledge of how to use it for a good purpose. Electioneering often boils down to luring people with fairy tales with the implicit message: 'Just vote for me and everything will be all right'. Consequently the politicians do not like to admit that there may be ills for which they have no painless remedies, and which will persist even if they are elected or re-elected. And if they propose unwelcome remedies, their rivals might outbid them by offering painless placebos. Nor do the media have much inclination to risk their popularity by sounding alarms about the need for unpleasant safeguards or remedies. They prefer to highlight tragedies which do not call for costly sacrifices from everybody. In view of these general human weaknesses, it would be unfair to put on the homosexuals all the blame for inaction in the face of Aids.

In their latest book[2] Masters and Johnson focus on the heterosexuals. It is the measure of the hyperaestesia surrounding this topic that the book was treated by some reviewers as sensationalist or outrageous. In fact it contains neither startling information nor radical proposals, and is written in a sober matter-of-fact style. Only some of the captions are slightly sensationalist. The view that non-sexual transmission (other than through injections or transfusions) is possible, is shared by many specialists. The authors do not say that it is likely in non-intimate contact. Their recommendations do not go beyond the need to test patients in hospitals and maternity clinics. They stop short of advocating mandatory abortions for women infected with Aids, which is one of the necessary measures to save the health service. In addition there are good ethical grounds for such a practice: too much emphasis is put on the right to parenthood but not enough on the right of the yet-to-be-born to a satisfactory life. If we have the duty to avoid actions which cause avoidable suffering, then nobody has a right to bring into the world a child known in advance to be condemned to a life of suffering without hope.

As an aside I must add that there are people who would like the National Health Service to disappear, and might even be glad that Aids is likely to put an end to it. They justify their attitude by invoking the superiority of market economy over a bureaucratised provision of goods and services. Despite being a firm partisan of market economy on the whole, I find this argument an example of how a good principle can be pushed to absurd lengths. Medical care is the field where social desirability of market mechanisms is the most questionable. Most goods and services will be wasted if they are given free of charge, because people will have no incentive to be economical: many will take more than their fair share and more than they can consume, while those who consume less than others will feel unjustly treated. Few people, however, have an unquenchable appetite for medical services. True, some people waste the general practitioners' time, but hardly anybody wants to have an unnecessary operation. There cannot be many taxpayers who resent being healthy and not getting their money's worth out of the Health Service. Moreover the market works best where the customer is able to try different products and judge their quality, which a patient is seldom in a position to do. Usually people need medical treatment most when they feel helpless and their judgement is impaired. They want to trust the doctor and such a trust helps recovery. So great abuses are likely when the quest for profit is the latter's sole motive. The State of California employs a team of detectives whose task is to catch doctors who give false diagnoses in order to profit from unneeded operations. And we must not forget that when the supply of anything depends on the market, the quantity and quality of what people get depends on their wealth. The Health Service is on the verge of collapse mainly because attitudes to life, sickness and death – within the medical profession as well as among the people and the politicians – have not been adjusted to the situation created by technical advances. In addition to sickness caused by pollution, Aids is likely to be the final blow. According to the latest American estimates, there will be 450,000 sufferers from Aids in the USA by 1993. A figure given for Edinburgh at the beginning of 1989 is 1 per cent of males aged 18–45.

The recent proposals to reorganise the National Health Service in Britain may have been prompted by the politicians' desire to pass downwards to the general practitioners the responsibility for making invidious decisions about allocating medical care which will not suffice for everybody. Moreover, a contraction of the public service will ensure that the rich will not suffer from the scarcity of medical resources.

Masters and Johnson's empirical study of heterosexual behaviour shows the connection between the incidence of infection and the number of sexual partners, which can be surmised on the ground of logic alone. Indeed it would be very puzzling if it were not the case. They also supply another confirmation of the tendency of homosexuals to change partners much more frequently on the whole than heterosexuals do. Given these two facts, the spread of the disease among heterosexuals ought to be much slower than it has been among homosexuals, if we relate the rate to the total numbers in each category. But there are sectors of the heterosexual population where partners are changed very frequently. There the spread might be just as fast as it has been among the homosexuals, albeit some difference might still remain in consequence of lesions, which are a common consequence of anal intercourse. According to Gene Antonio, many homosexuals have permanent suppurating sores around the anus. He also describes various sadistic practices among them which must cause even graver lesions.

Only in Africa are serious lesions of the vagina common, if not universal. I have already said earlier that female circumcision (which involves dreadful mutilations) might account for the un- paralleled speed of the spread of Aids in Africa. A recent article in *The Doctor* reports that the wounds from it are seldom completely healed and that most African women have permanent sores around the vulva. The report also maintains that this prompts a great deal of anal heterosexual intercourse. The latter point, however, is unimportant, because a vagina with sores is likely to be more vulnerable to infection than a healthy anus. If follows that nothing effective can be done to slow down the spread of Aids in Africa without first abolishing this cruel custom.

To my earlier remarks about widespread misuse of syringes, which I have observed in Nigeria, I must add that even the witch doctors (who treat many times more people than do scientifically-trained doctors or nurses) have added injections to their traditional procedures and give jabs with phoney medicines. They do not sterilise the needles.

I must also add a few words about syringes to my earlier remarks about the new dangers of imprisonment. According to a press report of a recent statement by a prison medical officer, contaminated syringes are widely used because they are smuggled in, concealed and shared . . . naturally without even the most rudimentary sterilisation. This is very serious, because the frustrations and despondency of prison life make relief through drugs particularly tempting, even to individuals who would keep well away from them when free.

Since the forecast was written, new grounds have appeared for suspecting that illicit experiments in genetic engineering may have been carried out in Africa. The first is the news about the dumping of toxic chemicals in Africa. If this can be done, either by agreement with governments or by bribing officials and duping ignorant property owners, then why not much less obtrusive and seemingly harmless experimentation? That there are companies who would do it is attested by the recent reports in the press about a pharmaceutical company which has been conducting in Argentina experiments in genetic engineering which are prohibited in Europe and North America. This experimentation was stopped when the Argentinian government was alerted by its scientists. In tropical Africa, the scientists are fewer while the governments are poorer and therefore more susceptible to financial enticements. For these reasons it would be the easiest target for illicit experimentation. Nevertheless, the plausibility of this explanation of the origin of Aids is weakened by the general argument put forth by the Harvard bacteriologist Bernard D. Davis whose book I have just read.[3] He makes the point that the number of human interventions through genetic engineering is exceedingly small in comparison with the number of recombinations of DNA occurring naturally every second. His second point is that existing strains of bacteria (and the same presumably applies to viruses) are products of long, constant and very severe natural selection, Artificial interference in the constitution, therefore, is practically certain to produce a less viable entity. These arguments, however, do not apply to experimentation through breeding, as in preparation for bacterio- logical warfare. The hypothesis that this might be the origin of Aids is even more radically weakened, if not refuted, by a report from Norway which appeared in the press recently.

In one of the hospitals in Norway they found samples of blood taken from a sailor who died in the nineteen-sixties from an illness which was not understood. His wife and child died a little later. Antibodies against HIV have been found in the samples. It was also discovered that this sailor spent some months in Africa in 1962, in the area now noted for the incidence of Aids. This was before the development of biotechnology. Therefore the other explanation is more likely to be correct. The anthropological report mentioned earlier about syringes being used to inject green monkey's blood into men's veins dates from 1972, but it is perfectly possible that the practice goes farther back in time. Syringes were available in central Africa before 1962.

The reports from the international congress about Aids held in Stockholm in June 1988 point in disparate directions. On the one hand, progress has been made in understanding the virus and towards the development of remedies, although nothing decisive has been achieved so far in the latter endeavour. On the other hand, the hopes have been dimmed by other findings. The increased understanding has revealed the extraordinary variability and 'cunning' of the virus. Already some time ago a variant called HIV2 was discovered in Africa. It now exists in Britain but the blood for transfusions is not screened against it. At the said congress it was reported that a new variant HIV3 has been discovered and that there may be intermediate forms, the same virus being able to assume different forms in response to differences in the environment. Another specialist maintains that the HIV2 virus can remain dormant for up to 20 years. I do not see how anybody can know this so soon after its discovery. But, if it is true, then the catastrophic effects of a snowballing spread might be even greater than hitherto feared, though they would occur after a longer delay. This is not the place (nor do I have the qualifications) to discuss the technical details. What matters most from the viewpoint of social consequences is that all the specialists agree that the ability of the virus to assume different forms makes it immensely difficult to devise a vaccine or a cure. Nevertheless, at the beginning of February 1989 an announcement came out that a new medicament has been produced – a genetically engineered molecule – which is expected to be more effective than the AZT without equally undesirable side-effects. However, like the AZT, it cannot cure but may be able to delay the onset of the illness. However, though of benefit to the unfortunate victims, medicaments incapable of exterminating the virus are likely to have undesirable side-effects on the collective level. The most obvious of them is an aggravation of the burden on medical resources. More important, however, would be a prolongation of the period of free circulation of the carriers which is likely to increase the number of new infections. To have a good effect on public health, a paliative would have to make the carriers uninfectious. If this were achieved, isolation would become entirely pointless, as the same result could be obtained by effectively enforced regular medication. In such a situation people would have much less reason to fear a test, but, to make sure that every carrier is being treated, obligatory testing might be necessary.

Another recent discovery discussed at Stockholm has revealed an additional difficulty of coping with Aids: namely that the virus can hide much longer than hitherto believed, remaining in the body for many months or even years without reproducing itself or provoking the production of antibodies. As this makes the tests less reliable, it has been argued that estimates of the infected must be revised upwards perhaps by a third. According to a recent press report, the testing of patients admitted to casualty departments in two hospitals located in poor areas of large cities in the USA has shown 5.3 per cent to be infected.

I have mentioned earlier that their readiness to resort to medico-social surgery may give close totalitarian systems an unexpected advantage. It remains to be added that any difference in the ability to check the spread of Aids will affect the balance of economic, political and military power. Among the rich nations, Japan appears to have the lowest incidence of Aids. Nevertheless, it is the most willing to adopt vigorous countermeasures. According to recent press reports, a law is being prepared for the Japanese parliament which will impose an obligation to submit to a test, if suspected of being a carrier, and to various restrictions on activities and movements, if found to be infected, with provision for close supervision. If these defences prove to be effective while other industrial nations procrastinate until they have to cope with many millions of sufferers, Japan's economic pre-eminence will attain new heights and may be followed by political influence and military power. If China is able to contain Aids better than the USSR, the balance of power between the communist giants might be reversed.

According to the recent reports, it has been decreed in the USSR that all foreigners coming for more than three months must be tested, and those infected will be debarred or deported. Nearly 200 foreigners have already been deported. All Soviet citizens returning after more than three months abroad must be tested. Every inhabitant suspected of being a carrier must submit to a test and, if infected, must collaborate with the medical authorities and the police who have the duty to trace and test all his or her sexual contacts. The reports do not make it clear what happens to the carriers. In Cuba, however, which has similar regulations about testing and the tracing of contacts, it has been officially confirmed that all known carriers are compulsorily interned. In Bulgaria (as I was told by a highly placed specialist) the government is planning compulsory testing of the entire population.

In contrast to Christian fundamentalism, Islamic revivalism is unlikely to impede the spread of Aids, because Islam imposes constraints only on women, while men are free to follow their impulses so long as they do not interfere with other men's wives or daughters. Adultery is conceived as a trespass against proprietorship. An important factor in the spread of Aids is the prevalence of homosexuality among the Moslems – the consequence of the cloistering of women and polygamy which enables rich men to corner the market for women while poor men are obliged to seek gratification with each other.

Despite the likely aggravation of the struggle for increasingly scarce medical resources, Aids will probably have a pacifying (or soporific) effect on internal politics because of a depletion of the young age cohorts which supply the majority of participants in violent actions. In electoral politics this depletion will entail a shift in favour of 'grey power' although the economic effect will be opposite: a stronger position of the workers because of their scarcity. This scarcity ought to provide an additional stimulus to automation. Internal peace is also likely to be promoted by the particularly high mortality of the slum-dwellers which will reduce the numbers of the discontented. For the same reason the crime rates will probably go down. Nevertheless this tranquillising influence on the social order might be counterbalanced, if not outweighed, by the spurring effects of increased sexual frustration.

Whereas the unemployed in the thirties demonstrated or rioted and supplied many recruits to communist or fascist parties proposing to overthrow the existing social order by violence, their counterparts today give little trouble to the rulers. A part of an explanation of this contrast is the much better provision of public assistance which in the rich countries prevents hunger and the lack of shelter or basic clothing. Nevertheless, life on public assistance is miserable enough (except perhaps in Australia or Sweden) to foster discontent and protest. So, there must be other factors involved. One of them is, no doubt, the soporific effect of addictive gaping at television, which is probably strong enough to account for the passivity of old-age pensioners who do not protest against their shabby treatment. The young adults, however, cannot be tranquillised so easily because they have more energy and spend less time in front of the box. The explanation of the political quiescence of the young unemployed seems to be that they expend their energy on revelry and fornication – the outlets which in the nineteen-thirties were available only to the sons of the rich. Radios and tape recorders can be obtained very cheaply secondhand, while contraceptive pills are inexpensive or can be obtained free of charge from a clinic. And practically everybody nowadays has access to a television set. So the young unemployed can make their impecunious existence quite entertaining by organising parties (where a few reefers are passed around), dancing and fornicating. The rest of the time can be filled with watching the 'telly', while even during the remaining intervals, serious thought or conversation is prevented by deafening pop music.

Religion may have functioned as 'the opium of the masses' in the past (as Marx and his followers have argued) but today this function is performed more efficiently by pop culture. In particular the cult of enormously wealthy pop stars must blunt somewhat the resentment which the poor normally feel against the rich. Because of its efficacity as opium of the masses, pop culture is welcomed by rulers who have to rely on manipulation rather than brute coercion. It is assiduously promoted even by state or semi-statal (like the BBC) radio and television, although being publicly financed they could well leave mere entertainment to the commercial networks, and devote themselves to the educational purpose of raising (or at least maintaining) the cultural and moral level of the population. Even communist governments began to understand the usefulness of pop culture for weakening political activism. In Poland – where their power is most precarious – pop festivals have been officially encouraged evidently to draw the young away from underground Solidarity which (because of its association with the Church) is slightly prim. Some festivals have been organised precisely on the days when Solidarity was planning demonstrations. A similar idea seems to have occurred to a tyrant in Ancient Greece who (according to Montesquieu) tried to prevent a rebellion by encouraging licentiousness among his potential opponents, sending to them beautiful courtesans.

The entire pop culture rests on the message of self-indulgence – especially in the matter of sexual novelty. But if the fear of Aids destroys its appeal, the young might seek an outlet for their energies in political action, perhaps mixed with religious issues – which would make the task of governing them much more difficult.

This applies not only to the unemployed but also to young workers (whether blue- or white-collar) in routine jobs, who find relief from utter boredom in sexual adventures wrapped up in pop culture. Bored as well as sexually frustrated, such people might be more eager than they are nowadays to join revolutionary movements of which ever colour might be in vogue at the time.

There is little doubt that sexual frustration stimulates aggression: most obviously and overtly in men but (though usually in a more indirect and covert way) also in women. An unformulated awareness of this connection may have underlain the practice (common in many tribes and states) of obliging warriors to abstain from intercourse while preparing for a campaign. In the Roman army it was three months. The soldier-monks were renowned for their combativity. In many armies soldiers were not allowed to marry – albeit here the most important consideration was to prevent permanent attachments: unattached men are not only more mobile but usually also readier to gamble with their lives. The janissaries lost their famous fighting qualities when the prohibition of marriage lapsed in the eighteenth century. The desperate sexual frustration of most young men may account (at least in part) for the violence and vindictiveness of Arab mobs whether in ethnic or revolutionary conflicts, as well as for similar aspects of the Iranian revolution. Owing to the absence of polygamy, there was no cornering of the market for women by the rich in Europe but nevertheless, in pre-permissive times most young men were sexually frustrated because they could not marry until they were able to support a family; many did not even have the money for a prostitute, while other young women were closely guarded. As the means of contraception will remain available, it is unlikely that the inability to support a family will again become the cause of men's sexual frustration. Nevertheless, the fear of disease may make the process of finding a partner much more laborious and lengthy, thus increasing the amount of sexual frustration in the society and thereby generating more aggressiveness. On the other hand, if the fear of infection prompts greater stability of marriages and brings down the number of abandoned, neglected or illegitimate children, it may reduce the amount of frustration of the basic needs for stability and security, which at present probably constitutes an important source of aggressiveness – particularly of the kind which finds an outlet in wanton violence and vandalism. What might be the balance of these opposite tendencies? My guess is that political activism and violence will increase but hooliganism and vandalism will decrease. But there is also another aspect ot the problem.

As you remember, Freud regarded sublimation of sexual desire as the source of all cultural creativity. As with most of his theses, Freud's insight seems valid up to a point, but exaggerated. As far as I know, nobody has attempted to assess its validity by a systematic survey of biographies of known contributors to culture. Did they differ in this respect from less creative individuals? A cursory glance at this material suggests that there are many cases which fit Freud's thesis perfectly (for example Isaac Newton, Immanuel Kant or Herbert Spencer), but others (like Bertrand Russell or Oscar Wilde) fit it less or not at all. On the whole it seems that Freud's thesis fits scientists and scholars much better than artists, novelists, poets and musicians, among whom there were many obsessive womanisers or pederasts.

A comparison of societies or historical periods throws an equally ambiguous light on Freud's thesis. The rise of Puritanism and the injection of some of its ingredients into the Catholic Church coincided with the birth of science and efflorescence of literature and the arts as well as a surge of business enterprise and geographical exploration. But the Italian Renaissance began well before Puritanism, while the Ancient Greeks – perhaps the most creative nation that ever existed – never knew anything even remotely resembling Puritanism, as even the stern Spartans engaged in public orgies.

Freud's thesis helps to explain the recent drying-up of creativity outside the natural sciences and technology, where inventiveness in the service of business and the armed forces has become institutionalised. In other fields there seem to be plenty of gimmicks but little true originality. This trend is particularly marked in the social sciences which have always suffered from their serviceability for propaganda, and which have largely succumbed to academic parasitism. More than a century ago Augustin Cournot doubted the feasibility of a science of politics because in this field, he said, 'it is inconceivable that telling the truth can ever become more profitable than telling lies.' Consequently, progress in the study of society depends not only on the available accumulated knowledge but also on the existence of idealism – a commitment to the search for truth regardless of personal advantage. Now, it is arguable that the hedonism of the permissive era is inimical to such idealism. It follows that a movement away from this hedonism might foster a revival of original thinking in this field. However, even if Freud's thesis were substantially valid, it would be rash to derive from it a firm forecast because there are many other factors involved: bureaucratisation, the bulldozing of cultural differences, and the stereotyping of minds by the mass media, may suffice to ensure cultural stagnation or even retrogression.

Aids might arrest (or even reverse) the population explosions in the poor South, but this will probably happen too late to prevent the turning of the rain forests into deserts. So, mass starvation and slaughter may increase even faster than the mortality from Aids. In any case, enough people will remain in the rich North (especially the affluent oldsters) to continue the destruction and poisoning of the environment. Coping belatedly with the disastrous and largely irreversible effects of pollution will probably be the chief preoccupation of mankind during the next century despite Aids.

Notes

1. *The Aids Cover-Up? – The Real and Alarming Facts About Aids*, Gene Antonio (second edn, with supplement: Ignatius Press, San Francisco, 1986).
2. *Crisis – Heterosexual Behaviour in the Age of Aids*, William H. Masters MD, Virginia E. Johnson and Robert C. Kolodny MD (London: Weidenfeld and Nicolson, 1988).
3. Bernard D. Davis, *Storm Over Biology* (Prometheus Books, Buffalo, 1986).

Index

Acquired Immune Deficiency
　Syndrome
　see Aids
Adler, Alfred, 188–9
Africa, 161
　Aids, 151, 165, 166, 179, 183, 184–5,
　　210–12
　attitude to women, 44–5, 183
　HIV virus, 184–5, 211–12
　syphilis, 6
　witchcraft in, 31–2, 41, 166
　see also Islam and Islamic lands
Aids (Acquired Immune Deficiency
　Syndrome), 20, 149–87, 203–18
　and entertainers, 171, 182
　and 'pop culture', 215–16
　and pornography, 171–2
　and sexual frustration, 215–17
　and xenophobia, 178, 179
　bisexuals, 169, 178, 181–2
　breakdown of health services, 166–8,
　　169, 209–10
　British Medical Association, 205–6
　carriers, 155, 157–8, 160–1, 167, 170,
　　178, 179, 180, 203, 204–5, 213,
　　214
　condoms, 154, 162–4, 165, 166, 167,
　　183, 203
　counselling, 156–7
　cure for, 153, 154, 181, 213
　drug addicts, 154, 166, 170, 171, 178,
　　211
　heterosexuals, 151, 165, 168–9, 178,
　　208–9, 210
　homosexuals, 157, 169–71, 178–9,
　　181–2, 203–4, 207–8, 210, 214
　in Africa, 151, 165, 166, 179, 183, 184–
　　5, 210–12
　in Britain, 149–51, 154, 166–9, 172,
　　203–7, 209–10, 212, 215–16
　in China, 179–80, 214
　in Germany, 179, 207
　in Japan, 160, 180, 214
　in prisons, 168–9, 211
　in USA, 157, 179, 180, 181, 184–5,
　　203–4, 213
　in USSR, 180, 183–4, 193, 214
　number of cases in UK, 149
　origin of, 151, 183–6, 211–12

physical elimination of sufferers, 164–
　5, 166, 180, 181, 182, 186, 213
reaction of British Government, 150–
　1, 154, 167, 172, 203–4, 210
religious revivalism and, 175–6
'safe sex' in age of Aids, 150–1, 203–
　4
scapegoats, 175, 177–8, 179, 207
segregation of sufferers, 157–64
should be notifiable disease, 206
suicide and euthanasia, 172
testing for, 155–6, 157–60, 162, 163,
　164, 204–6, 207, 209, 213, 214
transmission, 154–7, 209
Aids Cover Up?, The, 203, 207–8, 210
America, South, 125, 183
　conquered by Spain, 3–4
　Indians, 3, 7, 169
　syphilis spreads from, 5–7, 41–2
　see also USA
Antonio, Gene, 203, 207–8, 210
asceticism, 4–5, 8, 10, 13, 14, 17, 46, 177,
　198
Autoritaet Und Familie, 191–2
AZT (Aids drug), 213

Bacon, Francis, 21
Belgium
　commerce, 14–15
　Witch Hunts, 30
Bernard, Saint, 67, 68
bestiality, 30, 129, 133–5, 145
Beza, Theodore, 74
Bodin, Jean, 51, 65–6
Boguet, Henri, 92–7, 130
Borgias, The, (Popes), 5
Boyle, Robert, belief in witches, 21
British Medical Association, 205–6
buggery, 11, 168

Calvin, John, 5, 50
　and capitalism, 12–13, 26
　and puritanism, 12
　predestination belief, 15–16, 17–18,
　　26, 169
　Witch Hunts, 36, 37, 48, 74
Calvinism, *see* Calvin, John
capitalism, 13, 170, 200–1
　and Protestantism, 3, 14, 17, 18

220

226 *Index*

Trevor-Roper, Hugh, 23, 33
'*triage*' in treatment of Aids sufferers,
 167, 168
Trithemius, Abbot, 51
Turkey, syphilis in, 7–8

USA, 19
 Aids, 157, 179, 180, 181, 184–5, 203–
  4, 213
 conflict with USSR, 176
 doctors in, 209–10
 'McCarthyism', 37
 New England, 13, 50
 prohibition, 160
 religious revivalism, 177
 Second World War, 196–7, 199
 Witch Hunts, 50
USSR, 193
 Aids, 180, 183–4, 214
 conflict with China, 176
 Second World War, 197, 199
 Soviet agents in USA, 37
 Stalin, 34, 36, 195–7, 199
 syphilis in, 6, 7, 13
 Witch Hunts, 19, 48

Vanelli, Dr, Ronald, 37–8
venereal disease, 9, 10, 19, 58, 77, 80,
 163
 see also Aids, gonorrhoea, pox,
  syphilis

Wars of Religion, 11, 30–1, 33–4
Weber, Max, 3, 14, 16, 21
werewolves, 23
Weyer, Johannes, 60, 66
White, Andrew, D., 66–7, 70–5
*Witch-Cult In Western Europe. A Study In
 Anthropology*, 38–9
Witch-Finder General (Mathew
 Hopkins), 28
Witch Hunts and Witch Trials, 21–3, 150
 and Catholicism, 23, 36–7, 47–8, 81,
  90
 and Protestantism, 36–7, 47, 49
 and Wars of Religion, 33–4
 as persecution of pre-Christian
  religions, 38–9
 capitalism as factor, 25–7, 31–2
 celibacy as factor, 49, 59, 79, 81, 82
 change in attitude of church, 23
 children as victims, 35
 in England, 50

 in France, 26–7, 29–30, 44, 58, 61, 78,
  88
 in Germany, 26–7, 33, 35, 49, 58, 61,
  80
 in Holland, 26, 78
 in London, 27, 78
 in Luxembourg, 27
 in Poland, 27, 28
 in Scotland, 27, 30–1, 37, 49
 in Spain, 34
 in Switzerland, 27, 61, 79
 Lancaster Witches, 60–1
 male victims, 25, 30, 44
 manifestation of class conflict, 27–9,
  31, 81
 persecution of midwives, 80
 puritanism and, 19, 50, 79, 81
 role of Inquisition, 34, 35–6
 soldiers as victims, 30–1
 syphilis as cause, 18, 19, 41, 44, 57–
  9, 61–6, 75, 76–82, 150, 178, 190–
  1
 women as victims, 24–5, 28–30, 35,
  36, 38, 44, 80–2, 88, 150
Witch Hunters, 28, 30, 36, 87
 obsession with lust and disease, 51–
  9
 see also Boguet, Lancre, Remy, Witch
  Hunts
witchcraft, 21–2, 23, 24, 30, 34, 36, 87
 and celibacy, 88–91
 and lust, 51–9
 as an excuse for syphilis, 60–1
 as scapegoating mechanism, 37
 causes disease and illness, 32, 41, 51–
  2, 54, 59, 60–1, 65, 66–7, 68, 71–
  3, 82, 92, 96, 98–104, 109–12, 131
 causes impotence, 88
 in Africa, 31–2, 41, 166
witches, 21, 24, 33, 36, 61
 burning of, 34, 38, 47
 cause disease and illness, 32, 41, 51–
  2, 54, 59, 60–1, 65, 66–7, 68, 71–
  3, 82, 92, 96, 98–104, 109–12, 131
 church condemns belief in, 23
 interfere with procreation, 54–6, 66,
  92
 Lancaster Witches, 60–1
 sabbat, 23, 38, 87–8, 94–7, 126–7, 128–
  30, 136, 146
 sexual relations with incubi, 53–4, 95,
  105–8, 124–6, 129, 132–3, 135–41,
  143–6
 sexual relations with Satan, 93–6

witches – *continued*
  sexual relations with succubi, 53, 95, 105–8, 124–6, 129, 132–3, 135–41
  torture of, 28, 32, 34–5, 38–9, 73
  women as, 36, 51–9
  see also Witch Hunts, witchcraft
wizards, 136–41, 145–6
Wolsey, Cardinal, 9
women, 11, 50
  as witches, 36, 51–9
  demonisation of, 45, 47–8, 50, 65, 82

  in Africa, 44–5, 183
  in Islamic lands, 16, 25, 49, 76–7, 177, 194–5, 214
  in syphilis epidemic, 9, 44, 45, 60
  victims of Witch Hunts, 24–5, 28–30, 35, 36, 38, 44, 80–2, 88, 150
  see also nuns and nunneries

'Yorkshire Ripper', the (Peter Sutcliffe), 197–8
Young Man And The Harlot, The, 9